MAIN LIBRARY
STO

D1457507

616.2 Z188m   7140222
ZAVALA, DONALD C., 1923-
MANUAL ON EXERCISE TESTING

ALLEN COUNTY PUBLIC LIBRARY

FORT WAYNE, INDIANA 46802

You may return this book to any agency, branch,
or bookmobile of the Allen County Public Library.

MANUAL ON EXERCISE TESTING: A Training Handbook

By

Donald C. Zavala, M.D., F.A.C.P., F.C.C.P.
Professor of Medicine
Director of the Pulmonary Diagnostic Labs,
Department of Internal Medicine
College of Medicine
The University of Iowa
Iowa City, Iowa 52242

1985

Composed at the University of Iowa, Iowa City, Iowa 52242

Manual on Exercise Testing: A Training Handbook
© 1985 by Donald C. Zavala. Copyright under the International Copyright Union. All rights reserved. This book is protected by copyright. No part of it may be reproduced, stored in a retrieval system, or transmitted in any form or by any means, electronic, mechanical, photocopying, recording, or otherwise, without written permission from the copyright owner. Made in the United States of America. Press of The University of Iowa, Iowa City, Iowa 52242.

Printed in the United States of America.

Library of Congress Cataloging-in-Publication Data
Zavala, Donald C., 1923-
   Manual on exercise testing.

   Bibliography
   Includes index
   1. Exercise tests—Handbooks, manuals, etc.
   2. Pulmonary function tests—Handbooks, manuals, etc.
   3. Respiratory organs—Diseases—Diagnosis—Handbooks, manuals, etc.
   I. Title.
RC734.E87Z37   1985   616.2'004754   86-6977
ISBN 0-87414-042-0

Allen County Public Library
   Ft. Wayne, Indiana

7140222

CONTENTS

OUTLINE

PREFACE

This monograph represents my efforts to succinctly describe the technique of exercise testing in a clinical setting. By no stretch of the imagination is this an extensive work nor is it meant to be. This work is an outgrowth of the pulmonary disease fellowship program at the University of Iowa Hospitals and Clinics, Iowa City, Iowa, where my responsibility is to train our fellows in the concepts, applications, techniques, and interpretation of cardiopulmonary performance during exercise testing.

As a teacher and academician, I have taken the work of distinguished investigators in the field of exercise testing and attempted to put their findings into a pragmatic, easily understandable form - something that can readily be used. Currently there are two outstanding research groups in the North American continent who have made significant contributions to our understanding of exercise physiology. In the United States: Karlman Wasserman (Harbor-UCLA Medical Center, Torrance, CA) and his co-investigators consisting of James E. Hansen, Darryl Y. Sue, and Brian J. Whipp. In Canada: Norman L. Jones and E.J. Moran Campbell (McMaster University, Hamilton, Ontario). I do not wish to slight anyone else, since I am sure that there are others, however, I have personally visited these two exercise laboratories and found them to be superb centers for research and training.

I welcome comments from the readers which may prove to be extremely useful in future modifications and revisions of this text. Even so, I sincerely hope that the practical approach which I have taken will be helpful to physicians, doctorate candidates, and cardiopulmonary technicians in postgraduate training as well as those specializing in cardiac and pulmonary evaluations, industrial claims, sports medicine, and rehabilitation programs.

For additional reading, I strongly recommend the following two first-rate, authoritative books on exercise testing which I am sure will serve as state-of-the-art references for some time to come:

1. Wasserman K, Hansen JE, Sue DY, Whipp BJ: Principles of Exercise Testing and Interpretation. Philadelphia, Lea and Febiger, 1986.
2. Jones NL, Campbell EJM: Clinical Exercise Testing, 2nd Edition. Philadelphia, W.B. Saunders, 1982.

And finally, good luck to all of you who wish to improve your skills in exercise testing and interpretation!

Donald C. Zavala, M.D.
Iowa City, Iowa, U.S.A.

ACKNOWLEDGMENTS

This handbook would not have been possible without the fine diagnostic facilities provided here at the University of Iowa Hospitals under the directorship of John W. Colloton and the ideal academic environment created by Dr. Francois M. Abboud, Professor and Head of the Department of Medicine and Dr. Gary Hunninghake, Professor and Chief of the Pulmonary Division.

                                                                    DCZ

BOOK ORDER INFORMATION

All proceeds from this edition are being placed in a special account, Department of Medicine, The University of Iowa College of Medicine for the purpose of supporting research and educational activities related to the field of pulmonary diseases.

ORDERS (check, money order, or institutional purchase order) should be made out to:

Department of Internal Medicine

And sent to:

Administrator
Department of Internal Medicine
SE 311 GH
The University of Iowa
Iowa City, Iowa 52242 U.S.A.

SYMPOSIA ON EXERCISE TESTING AND INTERPRETATION

1. Every March and October by Karlman Wasserman, M.D., and colleagues. Apply by writing to Dr. Wasserman, Division of Respiratory Physiology and Medicine, LAC Harbor-UCLA Medical Center, A-15 Annex, 1000 West Carson Street, Torrance, CA 90509
2. Every March and October by Donald C. Zavala, M.D. Apply by writing to Dr. Zavala, Department of Medicine, Pulmonary Disease Division, University of Iowa Hospitals & Clinics, Iowa City, IA 52242

CHAPTER 1
EXERCISE PHYSIOLOGY:
Background Information

How Exercise is Measured[1]

FORCE (Newton or kilopond) is defined as the product of mass (kilogram) times acceleration (meter $\cdot$ seconds^2). WORK (joule or kilopond-meter), which requires the expenditure of energy, is the product of force times distance (meter). POWER is the amount of work performed in a given unit of time (work $\div$ time) and is measured in watts or kilopond-meters/minute. If a mass of 1 kilogram is raised 1 meter, the work performed is called a kilopond-meter (kpm) and can be expressed as kpm/min. Currently many physiologists use watts as the unit of work, however, it is important to know the conversion factor of 1 watt = 6.12 kpm/min since the literature is replete with exercise tests in which the power output is measured in kpm/min. Ergo, 50 watts is about 300 kpm/min.

Body Metabolism[2]

Skeletal muscle may be regarded as a machine whose fuel is the chemical energy of ingested food. Body metabolism involves the conversion of foodstuffs into energy. Oxygen (O_2) in the atmosphere crosses the air-blood interface in the alveoli of the lungs, and then is transported as oxyhemoglobin in red blood cells to its destination where the O_2 is released to the mitochondria of tissue cells. At the cellular level, oxidation of the substrate occurs with the production of energy, and at the same time the mitochondria give off carbon dioxide (CO_2). Thus, skeletal muscle gets its fuel from food and utilizes the O_2 for the combustion of that fuel.

The chemical energy of ingested food cannot be used directly by skeletal muscle. Instead, adenosine triphosphate (ATP) serves as the "energetic intermediary" and must be generated at the appropriate rate. If O_2 is used in the process of work (aerobic metabolism), then either carbohydrate

(CHO) or free fatty acids can be utilized as the energy substrate. Protein is not used except under conditions of starvation. The balance of the utilization of CHO and free fatty acids depends on the fitness of the subjects. With fitness, there is an increased ability to utilize free fatty acids for the work, thereby conserving the CHO stores. O_2 is used in the system and the end products are CO_2 and water (H_2O). If O_2 is not used in the process (anaerobic metabolism), then ATP still must be generated at the same rate in order for the work to continue. But under anaerobic conditions CHO is what Whipp terms the "obligatory substrate precursor" for the energy, and the end product is LACTIC ACID. To produce the same amount of ATP anaerobically as aerobically, the glucose utilization rate must be increased 18 times:

$$\text{1 molecule of CHO (glucose)} \xrightarrow{\text{Aerobic Conditions}} \text{36 ATP molec's} \rightarrow \text{WORK} \begin{array}{l} \nearrow CO_2 \\ \searrow H_2O \end{array}$$

$$\text{1 molecule of CHO (glucose)} \xrightarrow{\text{Anaerobic Conditions}} \text{2 ATP molec's} \rightarrow \text{WORK} \rightarrow \text{LACTIC ACID}$$

Note: 30% of the energy from the oxidation of fuels goes into useful work, and the remaining 70% goes into heat loss.

The rate of change of O_2 uptake in the fit subject is appreciably faster than in the unfit subject. This oxygen deficit can easily be met by energy stores (oxygen and hydrogen phosphate) in the fit person but not in the unfit person. The fit subject will perform 100 watts (600 kpm) of work with the production of CO_2 and H_2O, whereas the unfit person will do the same amount of work but at the price of producing lactic acid.

Anaerobic Threshold[2]

When the work rate reaches a certain value, called the "point of inflection" or the **anaerobic threshold,** oxygen uptake increases rapidly throughout the remainder of progressive exercise and the subject produces lactic acid. Shortly thereafter the work becomes intolerable. The anaerobic threshold (AT) is a *central issue* in exercise physiology and is defined as the highest work rate or O_2 uptake that can be maintained without an increase in blood lactate.[2-7] This work rate can be sustained by subjects volitionally for long periods of time under steady state conditions. The point at which lactate begins to increase in the arterial blood can be detected without having to sample the blood (p. 3). This finding is based on the recognition that the major buffer of lactic acid is the bicarbonate system. In fact, the bicarbonate system provides 90% of the lactic acid buffer:

$$NaHCO_3^- + \text{Lactic Acid} \longrightarrow \text{Na Lactate} + HHCO_3 \begin{array}{l} \nearrow H_2O \\ \searrow CO_2 \end{array}$$

The CO_2 in this equation does not come from metabolism but from the bicarbonate used in buffering, and therefore is in addition to the metabolic CO_2 output. Thus, a sudden increase in CO_2 (and ventilation) occurs at the anaerobic threshold.

With an increasing work rate, the ventilation ($\dot{V}_E$), and the CO_2 output ($\dot{V}CO_2$) increase linearly up to the point of anaerobic metabolism; thereafter they increase non-linearly. Also at the AT, a rise in the hydrogen ion concentration (acidosis) stimulates the chemoreceptors to provide an additional drive to ventilation over and above that of CO_2. Although there is a great spread in anaerobic thresholds among untrained subjects, the usual range is 50-60% of the maximal work rate,[4,6] with the lower limit of normal at 40% of the predicted VO2max.[7] Understandably, the AT can serve as an index of fitness with higher values in fit than in unfit persons.[3] In sedentary people the lower limit occurs at 50 watts (300 kpm) = 1.0 L/min O_2 uptake = walking 3 mph. With training, the AT can be raised to 90% of the maximal work rate, providing the individual is healthy. Patients with cardiovascular disease have very low anaerobic thresholds.

Estimation of Blood Lactate[2]

The maximal amount of blood lactate present during progressive exercise can be determined indirectly by obtaining an arterial blood gas sample at rest and again at the maximal work rate (WRmax). For every 0.9 miliequivalent (mEq) fall in HCO_3^- there is a 1.0 mM/L rise in lactate. For example, if the HCO_3^- is 24 mEq at rest and 18 mEq at maximal exercise then:

$$24 - 18 = 6, \text{ and } 6 \div 0.9 = 6.7 \text{ mM/L lactate}$$

Summary on Metabolism

For work of short duration, CHO is the preferred fuel (CHO is metabolised with a respiratory quotient [RQ] of 1.0), whereas fatty acid stores are increasingly utilized (RQ = 0.7) for work of long duration. There is a precise requirement for O_2 utilization during exercise. Oxygen utilization is a determinant of the work rate you can do. The greater the O_2 uptake by the subject, the greater the work rate he can perform. However, the physiologic cost of the same work rate by two individuals may be entirely different, since one may be producing lactic acid (which causes the ventilatory requirement to be excessively high) while the other person is still in aerobic metabolism. Therefore, the highest work rate without lactic acidosis (anaerobic threshold) is the most important determinant for the subject's capacity to perform sustained exercise.

3

However, if the work is progressively increased, then metabolic acidosis occurs by the conversion of pyruvate to lactate in the cells, which is promptly buffered by bicarbonate ion [HCO_3^-] with the release of CO_2.[8] The AT can be determined by nadirs which occur in the $\dot{V}_E/\dot{V}O_2$ (ventilatory equivalent for O_2), "R" ($\dot{V}CO_2/\dot{V}O_2$), and the $P_{ET}O_2$ (end-tidal O_2) as discussed on pages 40-41.

CHAPTER 2
Preparations for the Exercise Test

Indications for Exercise Testing

Almost invariably, diseases affecting the heart, lungs, circulation and blood will cause an abnormal response to exercise and, in addition, will indicate the body system involved. Although a positive result may be non-specific as to an exact diagnosis, there are some diagnostic uses such as in the myocardial ischemia, peripheral vascular disease, pulmonary thromboembolism, unfitness, psychogenic dyspnea, muscle phosphorylase deficiency and exercise-induced asthma.[1]

The Clinical Usefulness of Exercise Testing

(1) To quantitate the exercise capacity and anaerobic threshold of the individual (fitness).
(2) To evaluate unexplained dyspnea.
(3) To diagnose and quantitate exercise-induced asthma.
(4) To determine the factors (cardiac vs. pulmonary) which limit the patient's activity.
(5) To carry out industrial and sports evaluations.
(6) To determine the extent of impairment in disability evaluations and compensation cases.
(7) To formulate exercise prescriptions for safe reconditioning and to evaluate the effectiveness of rehabilitation.
(8) To follow responses to therapy in patients with cardiopulmonary disease.
(9) To help assess the extent and follow the course of interstitial lung disease, including response to therapy (e.g., steroid therapy in sarcoidosis).
(10) To help detect and follow iatrogenic pulmonary fibrosis caused by chemotherapy (e.g., bleomycin, methotrexate, myleran).

Contraindications for Exercise Testing

Nothing can replace sound clinical judgement. For review, a list of contraindications is provided here to alert the physician of potential, or outright dangerous situations which could cause serious harm to the patient under the conditions of stress testing:

(1) A poorly cooperative patient or one who is not capable of performing the test because of weakness, pain, fever, dyspnea, incoordination, or psychosis.

(2) Acute EKG changes of myocardial ischemia or serious cardiac arrhythmias including bradyarrhythmias, tachyarrhythmias, the sick sinus syndrome, and multifocal premature ventricular contractions. Occasional PVC's are not a contraindication.

(3) Congestive heart failure.

(4) Unstable angina.

(5) Recent myocardial infarction (within the first four weeks) or myocarditis.

(6) Aortic stenosis.

(7) Aneurysm of the heart or aorta.

(8) Severe pulmonary hypertension (cor pulmonale).

(9) Uncontrolled systemic hypertension, diabetes, arthritis, thyrotoxicosis, myxedema, asthma, or epilepsy.

(10) Acute thrombophlebitis or deep venous thrombosis.

(11) Severe electrolyte disturbances.

Evaluation of the Patient

Close adherence to a well worked-out program is the ideal way to approach exercise testing. Often it is useful to talk to the referring physician. Why was the test ordered? A questionnaire, check list or printed form similar to the one shown in Figure 1 is useful. The following pre-exercise work-up is recommended:

(1) **History and physical examination.** Remember to include occupation, exposure to noxious agents, degree of physical activity, habits (smoking, alcohol), diet, and medications. Specifically inquire about shortness of breath, wheezing, cough, sputum production and chest pain. Review any old chest x-rays or EKG's. Check the subject's weight, height, heart rate, blood pressure, heart tones, chest sounds, fingers for clubbing, and legs for edema.

(2) **Complete blood count and urinalysis.**

(3) **Spirometry.** FVC, FEV_1, FEV_1/FVC, and flow-volume loop. The subject's 15-sec MVV $\times$ 4 (1-min maximal voluntary ventilation) is used in calculating the ventilatory limit to exercise (pp. 39, 47, 52).

PRE-EXERCISE EVALUATION

NAME_____ AGE_____ SEX_____ HT_____ WT_____ DATE_____

REFERRING MD_____ OCCUPATION_____

REASON FOR REFERRAL_____

DIAGNOSIS_____

EKG_____ CHEST X-RAY_____

PHYSICAL ACTIVITY_____

SYMPTOMS: DYSPNEA_____ CHEST PAIN_____ WHEEZING_____

COUGH_____ SPUTUM_____ DIZZINESS_____

CLAUDICATION_____ OTHER_____

HISTORY: HYPERTENSION_____ HEART ATTACK_____ DIABETES_____

ARTHRITIS_____ ASTHMA_____ OTHER_____

SURGERY_____

MEDICATIONS_____

_____

MISCELLANEOUS_____

PHYSICAL
EXAM: BP_____ HEART RATE_____ HEART TONES_____

PERIPH. PULSES: CAROTIDS_____ RADIALS_____ PEDAL_____

CHEST_____

ABDOMEN_____

EXTREMITIES (clubbing, edema, veins)_____

NEUROLOGICAL_____

BONES AND JOINTS_____

COMMENTS: _____

_____

LAB CHECK-OFF LIST: CBC_____ UA_____ PFT's_____ ABG's_____ EKG_____ CXR_____

SIGNIFICANT LAB DATA_____

SIGNATURE_____

Figure 1. Pre-exercise evaluation.

In addition, the **measured** MVV can be compared with the **estimated** MVV (FEV$_1$ × 35-40); any major discrepancy should be investigated.

(4) Arterial blood gases (ABG's). An arterial sample is obtained pre-exercise, with the subject at rest, by needle puncture (blood gas kit) from the radial artery or occasionally from the brachial artery. A vital part of the test is to obtain another ABG at WRmax, just PRIOR to cessation of exercise. This maneuver is not difficult with the person on a bicycle, but is virtually impossible when the test is performed on a treadmill. Thus, when indicated, we use an arterial catheter, but the least invasive procedure necessary for testing is always preferable.

(5) EKG and chest x-ray.

Informed Consent

A primary prerequisite for stress testing is to thoroughly inform each subject regarding the exercise test protocol, as well as the objectives, the benefits, and the risks involved. This information is presented in an informed consent form (Figure 2) which the subject is required to read and sign before the test is begun. In fact, the risk to the patient performing an exercise test under the supervision of experienced personnel is very small. In 1971, Rochmis and Blackburn reported only one death per 10,000 patients studied and a mortality incidence (myocardial infarction, severe arrhythmia) of 2.4 per 10,000 patients, based on approximately 170,000 tests done in many laboratories across the country.[9]

Preparation of the Patient

General information:
(1) The last meal before the exercise should be light and should precede the test by at least 2 hours.
(2) Cigarettes, coffee, tea, carbonated beverages (e.g., Coke, Pepsi), and alcohol should be avoided prior to the test.
(3) Heavy exercise should not be performed earlier in the same day of the test.
(4) Properly fitting drawstring pants, buttoned shirts with short sleeves, and comfortable sneakers should be worn by the subject.
(5) Ideally, the room temperature should be 21°C–23°C (70°F–73°F) to minimize the effect of heat on the body during stress.

Preliminary procedures

One responsibility of the exercise technician is to see that the equipment is set up and working properly before the arrival of the patient. Other duties of a well-trained technician include:

8

CONSENT FOR EXERCISE TESTING

1. I will do an exercise test on a bicycle or on a treadmill to find out my degree of fitness and the nature and extent of any lung, heart, or circulatory problem.
2. The equipment will be demonstrated to me before I start the test.
3. The test will check the air (oxygen and carbon dioxide) I breathe out of my lungs while pedaling on the bike or walking on the treadmill. Also an EKG machine will tell the doctor about my heart beat, a cuff on my arm will measure my blood pressure, and clip on my ear will record the saturation of oxygen in my blood.
4. I will breathe through a mouthpiece held between my lips and teeth while I exercise, and a clip will be placed over my nose to stop any air from leaking through my nostrils.
5. In most instances, blood will be drawn from the artery in my wrist while I am at rest (before exercising) and again at the peak of exercise just before I quit the stress test.
6. Occasionally the doctor will have to put a soft tube into an artery in my arm so that a number of blood samples (usually 5 to 10) can be drawn while I exercise.
7. There is no risk at all in the breathing measurements, and there is very little risk in the exercise test. If I have heart disease, the test could cause chest pain or irregular beats of the heart. The presence of the doctor at my side checking the blood pressure, watching the EKG machine, and following the saturation of oxygen in my blood make these risks as small as possible. If I have chest pain, irregular heart beats, dizziness, fall in blood pressure or drop in my blood oxygen, the doctor will take appropriate action.
8. During exercise, the work load will be increased steadily until I can go no further. On the other hand, I may stop anytime I don't feel right, or my doctor may tell me to stop the test.
9. After the exercise I probably will have sore, stiff muscles. Very rarely (never in our experience) will infection or clots appear at the site where blood (by needle or thin tube) was taken from the artery in my arm. If this happens, I will need further medical or surgical treatment.
10. I fully understand why this test is being done. I also know how it will be done and the extent of the risks. I agree to do the exercise test as described and realize that more than one exercise may have to be done.

DATE＿＿＿＿＿ PATIENT'S NAME ＿＿＿＿＿＿＿＿＿＿＿＿

HOSPITAL NUMBER＿＿＿＿＿

PATIENT'S SIGNATURE＿＿＿＿＿＿＿＿＿＿ (Parent if a minor)

DOCTOR'S NAME ＿＿＿＿＿＿ SIGNATURE ＿＿＿＿＿＿

Figure 2. Consent for exercise testing.

9

(1) wrapping the blood pressure cuff (mercury manometer) on the subject's upper arm;
(2) attaching the 12-lead EKG and 3-lead cardiotachometer;
(3) securing the oximeter to the ear (we use a Biox IIA and attach the probe to either the antihelix of the ear or the ear lobe);
(4) applying the noseclip tightly enough to avoid an airleak;
(5) positioning the mouthpiece correctly;
(6) showing the patient how to pedal the bicycle or to mount the treadmill. Familiarizing the patient to unaccustomed surroundings and equipment will help tremendously to reduce anxiety and to gain his or her confidence and cooperation.[10] Several trials on the cycle or treadmill may be necessary before the patient feels comfortable. At least one of the preliminary trials should be conducted with the mouthpiece and noseclip in place. If on the bicycle, the patient should practice at 50-60 rpm with a low resistance load. If on the treadmill, an easy walk-rate at zero elevation is used.

Electrode Placement

The Electrocardiogram

Satisfactory EKG tracings are much easier to obtain when the patient is on the cycle rather than the treadmill because of less "noise." We prepare the skin by rubbing the selected area with a Scotch-Brite pad (3M), then wiping thoroughly with alcohol, followed by dry gauze. Electrode placement in our laboratory is similar to that used by Wasserman (Harbor-UCLA Medical Center, Torrance, CA):

RA = Right supra-scapular area.
LA = Left supra-scapular area.
RL = Lower rib cage, anterior axillary line, right side.
LL = Lower rib cage, anterior axillary line, left side.
V_1-V_6 = All electrodes are placed across the chest on a line level with the 5th interspace.
V_1 = Right sternal border.
V_2 = Left sternal border.
V_3 = Midway between V_2 and V_4.
V_4 = Midclavicular line.
V_5 = Anterior axillary line.
V_6 = Midaxillary line.

The Cardiotachometer

Electrode placement is as follows:

RA = Posterior lower neck, just to the right of C-7.
LA = Just to the left of LL limb lead.

RL =   Just to the right of RL limb lead.

Note: Be sure to fasten cables with a sling to prevent movement. For obese patients, EKG electrode placement is the same; however, for the cardiotachometer, two of the three electrode placements (LA and RL) are changed: LA = Left infrascapular area; RL = right infrascapular area; RA = remains the same, i.e., on the posterior neck to the right of C-7.

CHAPTER 3
EXERCISE EQUIPMENT

Milieu

A temperature-controlled room (21°-23°C) with known relative humidity and adequate space for equipment and personnel is essential (Figures 3a, b, c). The area should have an ample number of separate, electrical outlets and a secure place for gas cylinders.

Shopping List

A semiautomated or fully automated exercise system will reduce errors and greatly speed up the display, printing, and storage of data. The following equipment is required for carrying out the procedures described in this monograph:

(1) Cycle ergometer, electromechanical
(2) Treadmill, motor-driven
(3) Mass spectrometer or rapid responding O_2 gas analyzer (e.g., fuel cell type)
(4) Mass spectrometer or rapid responding CO_2 analyzer (infrared type)
(5) Multichannel analog to digital (AD) converter and CRT (cathode ray tube) screen for display of data
(6) Breath-by-breath analyzer (otherwise a mixing chamber)
(7) Multiple lead EKG and cardiotachometer
(8) Pneumotachograph with differential pressure transducer
(9) Ear oximeter
(10) Computer (protected by a voltage regulator)
(11) Printer (hardcopy or teletype)
(12) Valves
(13) Gas cylinders: O_2 for the patient; O_2 and CO_2 mixtures for standardization of the gas analyzers

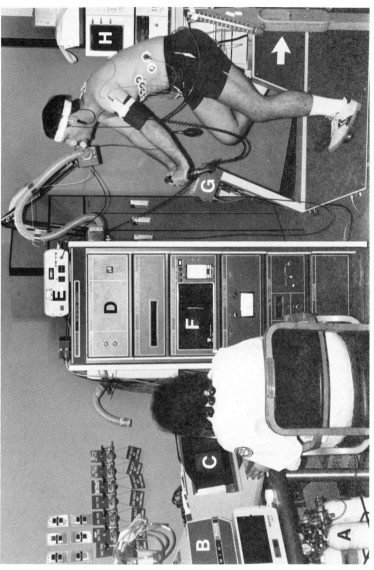

Figure 3a. **Medical Graphics Exercise System** in the Cardiopulmonary Exercise Laboratory at The University of Iowa Hospitals and Clinics: (A) gas cylinders for calibration of O_2 and CO_2 analyzers; (B) Tektronix 4631 hard copy unit; (C) Tektronix 4052 computer (Beaverton, OR); (D) MGC Exercise System 2000 (Medical Graphics Corp., St. Paul, MN); (E) Biox II ear oximeter (Ohmeda, Boulder, CO); (F) MGC visual display of EKG rhythm strip (easily viewed by the technician); (G) Kem-3 cycle ergometer; (H) Hewlett-Packard cardioscope model 78304A for continuous display of leads II, AVF, and V-5 on the CRT screen; a Hewlett-Packard EKG model 1505A is sitting on top. White arrow points to a sphygmomanometer with inflatable arm cuff. For accuracy, the blood pressure is taken manually.

13

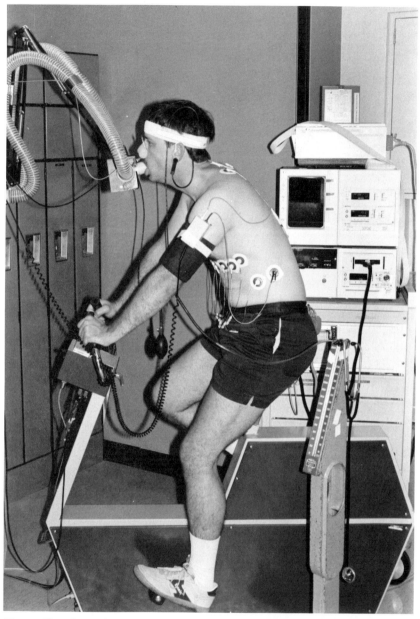

Figure 3b. View of the cyclist during the 2-minute rest period just prior to unloaded pedalling. A protective, mesh vest has been removed to show the EKG leads.

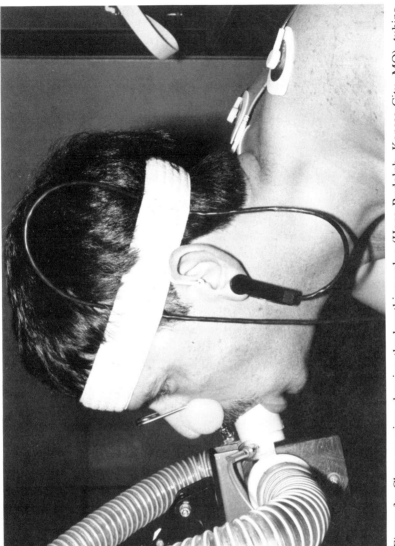

Figure 3c. Close-up view showing the breathing valve (Hans Rudolph, Kansas City, MO), tubing, mouthpiece, noseclip, headband, and oximeter probe (Biox IIA, Ohmeda, Boulder, CO) attached to the pinna of the ear. An alternate site for the ear probe is the anti-helix.

(14) Mercury manometer with blood pressure cuffs for normal-weighted and obese patients
(15) Blood gas analyzer
(16) Hygrometer-Thermometer
(17) Crash cart with cardiac defibrillator, manual resuscitation bag, intravenous sets, and emergency drugs
(18) Miscellaneous: mouthpieces, nasal cannulas, Douglas-type bags or balloons, tubing, connectors, three-way stopcocks, small syringes, calibration syringe (1.0 or 3.0 liter), blood gas kits, and arterial catheter setups

Purchasing Equipment

A bit of advice:

There are advantages to purchasing a computerized exercise system rather than trying to build your own. Extensive technical knowledge is required to assemble the equipment yourself and to write a rather complex software program. From an economic standpoint, one can investigate buying a complete exercise system as a single package or starting with the purchase of a basic unit to which the peripheral devices are added (e.g., treadmill, cycle ergometer, EKG, cardiotachometer, and ear oximeter). If money is no factor, then the ultimate in gas analyzers is to have a mass spectrometer, used in combination with a breath-by-breath analyzer. A less costly, but excellent setup, is to use rapid gas analyzers (O_2 and CO_2) in place of a mass spectrometer. The least expensive exercise system is the incorporation of O_2 and CO_2 gas analyzers with a mixing chamber. One should be aware, however, that difficulties may be encountered with mixing chamber systems in measuring rapid, dynamic changes in F_EO_2 and F_ECO_2 during incremental or ramp exercise.

There are several ways to interpret the meaning of the phrase "breath-by-breath", so when investigating the different types of "breath-by-breath" exercise systems, make certain that the following conditions are present: (1) The response time of the analyzers (O_2 and CO_2) is faster than 150 ms, measured from the subject's mouth to the sensor; (2) The flow signal is sampled at least 100 times per second or greater (if a volume transducer, then find out how fast the volume signal is sampled and differentiated ... to get flow); (3) The end-tidal O_2 and CO_2 values are displayed at the same time as the $\dot{V}O_2$ and $\dot{V}CO_2$; (4) The measured parameters are displayed in real time on the CRT screen immediately after each breath. In addition, there should be a way to accurately measure the time delay between the instantaneous flow signal and the time delayed gas signals (for use in computing the volume of gas in each breath). This computation requires a continuous flow signal and rapid response gas analyzers for O_2 and CO_2.

Manufacturers and Distributors

Cardiopulmonary Exercise Testing Systems
Medical Graphics Corporation (Figure 4a)
350 Oak Grove Parkway
Saint Paul, Minnesota 55110
Telephone 612/484-4874
1-800-328-4137 (Service)
1-800-328-4138 (Sales)

SensorMedics Corporation (Figure 4b)
1630 South State College Blvd.
Anaheim, California 92806
Telephone 714/634-0233

Gould Incorporated (Figure 4c)
Cardiopulmonary Products Division
805 Liberty Lane
Dayton, Ohio 45449
Telephone 513/859-9000

Erich Jaeger, Incorporated (Figure 4d)
5251 Zenith Parkway
Rockford, Illinois 61111-2728
Telephone 815/633-6400

Cybermedic, Incorporated (Figure 4e)
P.O. Box 3468
Boulder, Colorado 80307
Telephone 303/666-9253

Treadmills and/or Cycle Ergometers
Quinton Instrument Company (Figure 5a)
(Division of A.H. Robbins Company)
2121 Terry Avenue
Seattle, Washington 98121-2791
Telephone 206/223-7373
1-800/426-0337 (Sales)

Marquette Electronics, Incorporated (Figure 5b)
8200 West Tower Avenue
P.O. Box 23181
Milwaukee, Wisconsin 53223
Telephone 414/355-5000

Warren E. Collins, Incorporated (Figure 5c)
220 Wood Rd.
Braintree, Massachusetts 02184
Telephone 617/843-0610

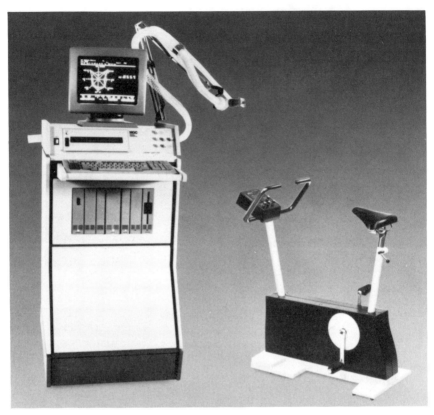

Figure 4a. **The Medical Graphics Corporation CAD/Net TM Cardiopulmonary Exercise Stress Testing System 2001** with a Kem-3 cycle ergometer. This system provides state-of-the-art, breath-by-breath analysis by measuring over 150 variables on every breath, including $\dot{V}O_2$, $\dot{V}CO_2$, $\dot{V}_E$, HR and their derivatives. Other features are rapid-response gas analyzers, linear flow transducer, high-performance 16-bit computer (Convergent Technologies, San Jose, CA), high resolution display monitor, disk storage of data, and rapid display of the test results in graphic and tabular form.

Ear Oximeters

Ohmeda (Figure 6a)
4765 Walnut Street
Boulder, Colorado 80301-2549
Telephone 303/447-9842

Nellcor Incorporated (Figure 6b)
25495 Whitesell Street
Hayward, California 94545
Telephone 415/887-5858

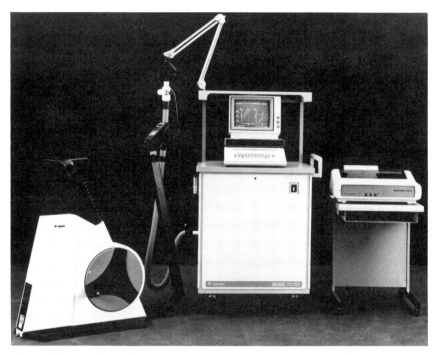

Figure 4c. **The Gould 9000 IV Computerized Pulmonary Exercise Lab** with a Lanooy-type bicycle ergometer. Computer choices include the Gould Workstation, the IBM-PC family, or the Convergent Technologies N-Gen. The system uses a "volume delay factor" which automatically corrects for the phase lag between volume and gas analysis. Hardware and other features include indirect cardiac output capability, dry rolling seal spirometer, paramagnetic O_2 analyzer, infrared CO_2 analyzer, graphic and tabular reports and the interface capability for up to 9 external devices.

Valves

A number of different valves with various dead space volumes and resistances are available, e.g., Otis-McKerrow, Lloyd, Koegel, Rudolph, etc.[1] Unfortunately, there is a trade-off between dead-space volume and resistance: the smaller the dead space, then the higher the resistance. Low dead-space valves are desirable, especially for accurate measurement of V_D/V_T, but one must be careful that the resistance is not too high. Generally a valve with a dead-space volume of 60-90 ml in adults is acceptable for clinical testing.

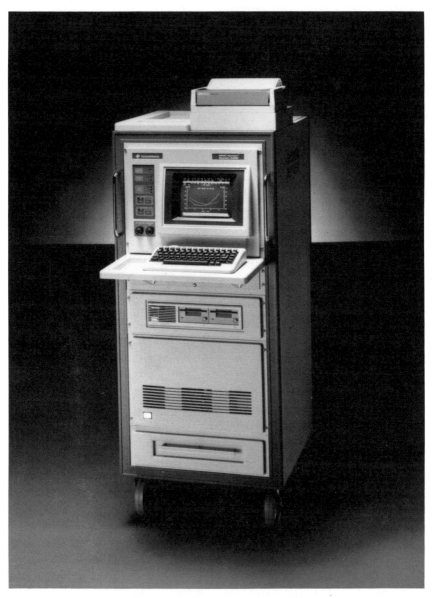

Figure 4b. **The SensorMedics MMC Horizon System 4400** which can be combined with the **ECG Horizon System** for complete cardiopulmonary stress testing, either on a bicycle ergometer or a treadmill. The MMC Horizon System 4400 consists of a 16/32 Bit H-P scientific computer with an internal memory of 512 Kbytes, digital volume transducer (turbine), electrochemical zirconium dioxide O_2 analyzer, infrared CO_2 analyzer, a breath-by-breath sampling system, and tabular and graphical displays of the test data.

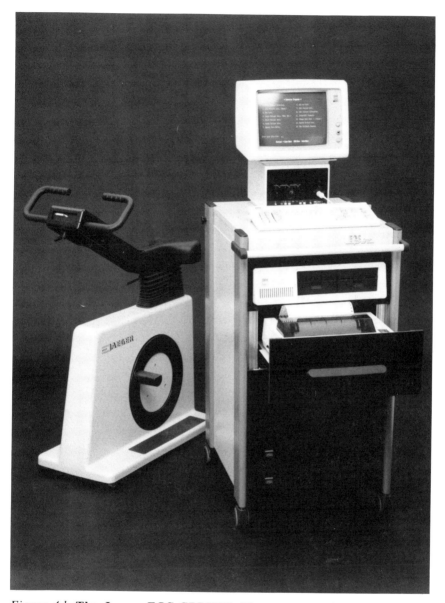

Figure 4d. **The Jaeger EOS SPRINT.** The setup consists of a mobile cardiopulmonary stress/metabolic testing system with O_2 and CO_2 analyzers, self adjusting mixing chamber, highly linear pneumotach, color CRT and printout, and a cycle ergometer.

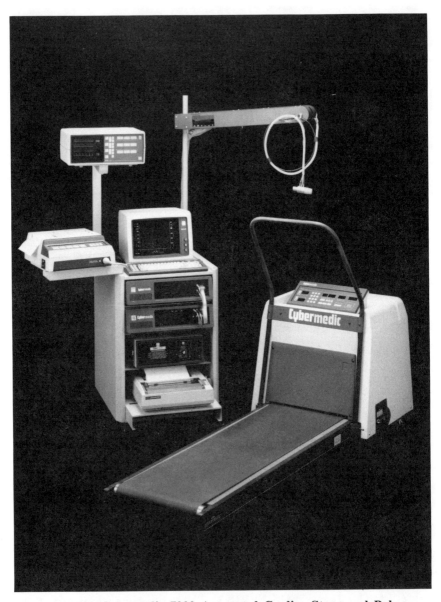

Figure 4e. **The Cybermedic 7000 Automated Cardiac Stress and Pulmonary Analysis System.** The equipment features a patented isowave waveform alignment, full color graphic display of metabolic parameters, and reports. A heavy duty programmable treadmill and EKG monitor also are shown in this photograph.

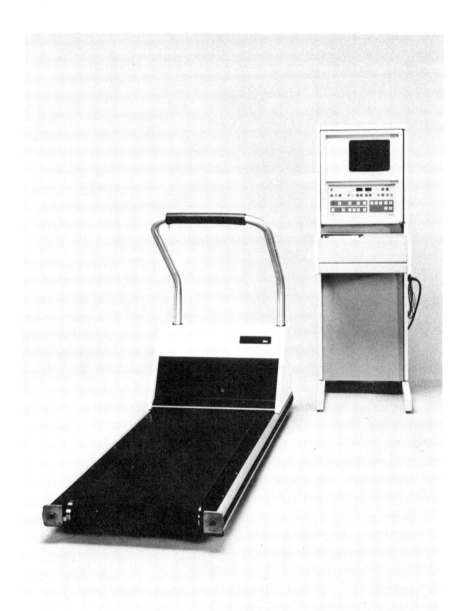

Figure 5a. **The Quinton (A.H. Robbins) Q-3000 Stress Monitor with the Q-55 Treadmill.** Attractive features include EKG monitoring, CRT display of data, and a tabular final report. The Q-55 treadmill has a 350 lb. capacity, a speed range of 1-10 mph, and a grade range of 0-25%. Up to 9 treadmill protocols can be programmed.

Mouthpiece

A persistent problem in exercise testing is the mouthpiece. Several difficulties may be encountered: (1) failure of some patients to obtain a tight seal with their mouth, especially the pediatric age group, the elderly and those with improper fitting dentures; (2) collection of saliva on the floor of the mouth and in the mouthpiece; (3) inability of the subject to swallow or to talk; (4) dry throat; (5) jaw fatigue from biting down on the mouthpiece. Currently a new type of mask is being developed by the author and Hans Rudolph (Kansas City, MO) which should circumvent these problems.

Breath-by-breath Analyzer vs. Mixing Chamber

The breath-by-breath analyzer, compared to a mixing chamber, has definite inherent advantages.[11,12] The computerized, breath-by-breath system provides rapid graphic and tabular display of extensive data and important interrelationships of selected measurements that help greatly in the interpretation of exercise performance. Other paramount advantages are: (1) measurement of end-tidal oxygen ($P_{ET}O_2$) and end-tidal carbon dioxide ($P_{ET}CO_2$), which facilitates identifying the anaerobic threshold; (2) increased accuracy during rapid changes in ventilation; (3) almost instantaneous display of data from each breath which is useful in quick evaluation of the patient from moment to moment rather than minute to minute. The amount of data shown immediately after each breath varies according to the software programs written by the various manufacturers. In most instances the following data are displayed: $\dot{V}_E$, $P_{ET}O_2$, $P_{ET}CO_2$, $\dot{V}O_2$, $\dot{V}CO_2$, R, HR, and O_2/HR. Options include the addition of V_T, f_b (RR), $\dot{V}_E/\dot{V}O_2$, $\dot{V}_E/\dot{V}CO_2$, and O_2sat%.

Treadmill vs. Cycle Ergometer

Treadmill

These motor-drive instruments were developed in North America by scientists who were interested in the field of work and sports physiology.[13] Originally treadmills were large, heavy, noisy, and expensive. Currently, many of these undesirable features have been modified or improved upon, although some disadvantages still remain. Upon making comparisons with a cycle ergometer, the following differences are unique to the treadmill: (1) cost, in some instances, is still a factor; (2) there is danger of a fall in spite of handrails; (3) the subject cannot stop exercising on his own but must continue walking as long as the belt is running or else fly off the end of the machine; (4) the power output (work rate) cannot be measured, although an estimation can be made from an equation based on body

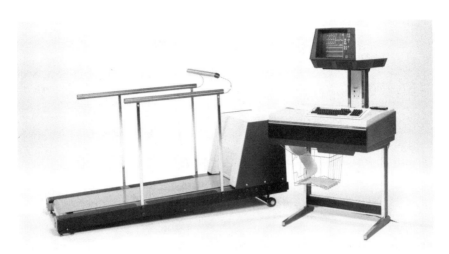

Figure 5b. **The Marquette CASE 11.** This monitoring unit is combined with a Series 1800 treadmill to give a complete EKG and stress testing system. A high resolution CRT is mounted on a swivel pedestal for easy viewing of ST-segment displacement (12 leads), arrhythmias, and other monitored parameters. A thermal printer is utilized for a comprehensive final report. A microprocessor (in the cable junction box) is used to help eliminate electrical interference and baseline wandering. A convenient feature is an infrared, hand-held remote control.

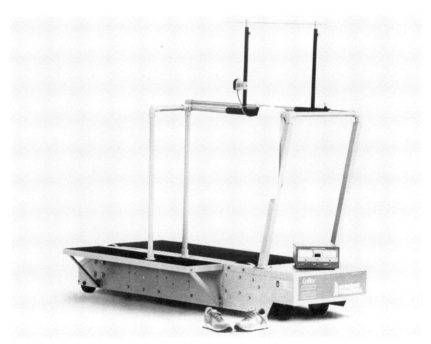

Figure 5c. **The Collins Treadmill.** The standard models (007205 and 007011) feature a 2 HP motor capable of producing speeds of 1-9 mph. The high speed model (007203) has a 5 HP motor with a speed range of 2-16 mph. EKG monitoring is not included.

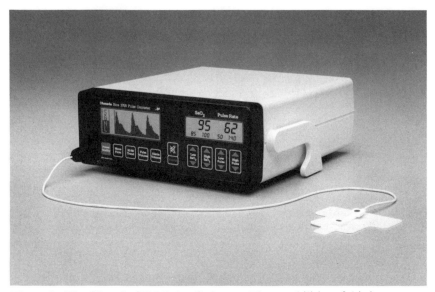

Figure 6a. **The Ohmeda 3700 Pulse Oximeter.** The capabilities of this instrument include continuous, non-invasive SaO$_2$% and pulse rate monitoring, plethysmographic waveform display, and an 8 hour Trend Memory of the SaO$_2$% and pulse rate data.

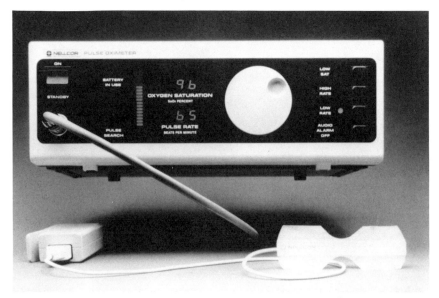

Figure 6b. **The NELLCOR N-100 Pulse Oximeter.** This instrument is an accurate, non-invasive device for measuring arterial oxygen saturation (SaO$_2$%) and pulse rate.

weight, speed and grade. Thus, performance on the treadmill is expressed in speed and inclination (grade) and not in kpm or watts; (5) blood pressure measurements (arm cuff), EKG recordings, and arterial blood gas samples (without cannulation) are more difficult to obtain than on a bicycle; (6) the response to a given work rate varies directly with the subject's weight, ergo, there is a higher $\dot{V}O_2$max when compared to a bicycle by 10%, a higher O_2/pulse by 6%, a larger stroke volume by 5%, and a greater A-V O_2 difference.[13]

These comments are not meant to imply that the treadmill is not a useful machine in clinical medicine. In fact, approximately 75% of the stress tests performed in America are on a treadmill.[14]

Cycle Ergometer

Bicycle ergometers were developed in Europe where researchers started with mechanical models, changing later to electromagnetic ones which allowed accurate measurement of resistance (power) in precise units (watts or kpm).[13] With electromagnetic resistance, the fly wheel moves through an electromagnetic field, and the strength of the field determines the resistance to pedalling. A constant level of work is maintained independent of the pedalling rate (40 to 80 rpm). A feedback loop increases the resistance when the rate slows, and decreases the resistance as the rate increases. In addition to accurate measurement of power, there are other advantages of a cycle over a treadmill: (1) the models are generally less expensive, lighter, portable, take up less room, and make no noise; (2) there is less danger of a fall; (3) the subject can stop exercising any time by choice; (4) it is easier to obtain blood pressure readings, EKG tracings and arterial blood gases (by radial artery puncture); (5) the results are independent of body weight since the subject is supported by a seat; (6) exercise can be carried out on patients in a recumbent position, e.g., during cardiac catheterization; (7) arm cranking, rather than leg pedalling, can be performed.

There are, however, some disadvantages to using a cycle: (1) the seat can be very uncomfortable, especially for overweight subjects; (2) exercise is limited more by muscle fatigue in the legs than by overall cardiovascular, respiratory, and metabolic fatigue; (3) some patients do not know how to ride a regular bicycle and are so poorly coordinated that cycling (even with training) is impossible for them.

Ear Oximeter, Blood Gas Kits, Arterial Catheters

To facilitate the evaluation of gas exchange dynamics, we routinely use a simple, non-invasive approach by continuously monitoring SaO_2% with a Biox IIA ear oximeter. Recently the Biox IIA ear oximeter was replaced by the newer Ohmeda Biox III (Ohmeda, Boulder, CO) as shown in Figure

6a. In addition to **ear** oximetry, the newer instruments made by Ohmeda and Nallcor (Fig. 6b) can accurately carry out **pulse** oximetry with the probe attached to the index finger. Also blood gas kits are used to draw an arterial blood gas sample from the radial artery prior to and near the end of exercise. Arterial blood sampling with the patient on the bicycle is not especially difficult but does require practice to become proficient. Thus, arterial oxygen desaturation can be readily detected at any time during the test,[15] and the arterial blood gas values, $P(A-a)O_2$, $P(a-ET)CO_2$ and V_D/V_T can be accurately measured at rest and at maximal work rate (WRmax). In selected cases, however, one may elect to insert a 5F polyethylene catheter into the brachial artery by the Seldinger technique[16] or to insert a teflon Becton-Dickenson "long dwell" catheter over a needle into a brachial or radial artery.[10] In this manner, blood gas samples (usually 5-10) and the blood pressure can be constantly monitored.

28

CHAPTER 4
EXERCISE PROTOCOLS

The Exercise Team

In a clinical setting, the exercise team usually consists of two persons, the physician and the technician. If possible, it is advisable to have another equally-trained physician and technician to serve as a backup if a member of the first team is absent.

The physician is responsible for:
(1) having a basic knowledge of exercise physiology (excellent exercise seminars are available periodically in several medical centers in the United States)
(2) carefully evaluating the patient prior to testing
(3) knowing the indications and contraindications for exercise testing
(4) obtaining an informed consent to perform the test
(5) observing the patient closely during exercise
(6) giving encouragement to the patient for a good performance
(7) taking the blood pressure every minute during exercise and also in the immediate post exercise period
(8) being aware of the HR, EKG tracing, SaO_2%, $\dot{V}_E$, $\dot{V}O_2$, and R values as the exercise progresses
(9) knowing when the patient is nearing exhaustion
(10) knowing when the exercise should be terminated prematurely
(11) drawing arterial blood gas samples at appropriate times
(12) making certain that the patient has a "cool-down" period immediately following exercise (1-2 minutes of unloaded pedalling or walking the slowest speed on the treadmill)
(13) checking the heart and lung sounds in the immediate post recovery period
(14) following the EKG and BP in the recovery period
(15) being well-trained in cardiopulmonary resuscitation

29

(16) supervising the exercise laboratory and performance of the personnel

The exercise technician is responsible for:
(1) pulmonary function testing
(2) drawing the arterial blood gas sample or assisting the physician in obtaining a specimen
(3) blood gas analysis
(4) carrying out quality control
(5) familiarizing the patient with the equipment before exercise, especially how to pedal the cycle or to mount and walk on the treadmill (At least one trial of mild exercise should be done with the noseclip and mouthpiece in place.)
(6) calibrating and operating the exercise system, including entry of patient information, barometric pressure, room temperature, etc., into the computer before exercise
(7) informing the doctor of pertinent values (e.g., HR, $\dot{V}_E$, $\dot{V}O_2$, R) as they appear on the CRT screen during exercise (It is important for the doctor to know when the "R" [$\dot{V}CO_2/\dot{V}O_2$] rises above 1.0 [p. 43].)
(8) disconnecting the patient from the equipment when finished
(9) compiling the computerized test data and graphs after exercise for interpretation by the doctor
(10) disinfecting the mouthpiece, valve, and tubing after each test
(11) turning off various pieces of equipment (note: the O_2 fuel cell is always left on) when the test is completed
(12) being well-trained in cardiopulmonary resuscitation

Treadmill Exercise Protocols

Generally, one of four types of treadmill exercise routines are employed, depending upon the nature of the subject's disability.

The Naughton Test.[17]

There are 10 exercise periods of 3 minutes, each one separated by 3 minutes of rest. After walking level at 1.0, 1.5 and 2.0 mph, the incline is increased to 3.5% and then to 7% at 2 mph. At the sixth period the speed is increased to 3 mph and the grade reduced to 5%; thereafter the grade is incremented by 2.5% each period and the speed held at 3 mph.

The Balke Test[18]

The speed remains at 3.3 mph, and the grade, starting at zero % for the first minute, increases by a 1% increment every minute. In the modified Balke test the belt speed remains at 3 mph, and the grade is increased 2.5% every 2 minutes.

The Fox Test

The belt speed stays at 3 mph, and the grade is increased 2% every 2 minutes.

The Bruce Test[19,20]

The speed and grade are increased every 3 minutes: 1.7 mph at 0%, 5% and 10% grade, 2.5 mph at 12% grade, 3.4 mph at 14% grade, 4.2 mph at 16% grade and 5.0 mph at 18% grade. Thereafter, the speed is incremented 0.5 mph.

The Jones and Campbell Test[1]

The speed stays constant at 2.0, 2.5, 3.0 or 3.5 mph, and the grade is increased 2.5% every minute.

Walking the Treadmill

Walking is a simple, natural skill practiced daily in our ordinary activities. Nevertheless, patients must be shown how to walk on the moving belt of a treadmill. To mount the treadmill, the first maneuver for the patient is to straddle the belt while holding onto the support bars. Next, the treadmill is started at its lowest speed (1.0 to 1.5 mph) and zero% grade. Then the left foot is placed on the belt and moved as though pushing a scooter. When ready, the patient steps on the belt and begins walking upright while looking straight ahead. At this point, most subjects can walk without holding the guard rails, however, this feat is not always possible. Not uncommonly, hospitalized patients prefer to rest at least one hand lightly on the guard rail for reassurance.

Riding the Cycle

The handle bar and seat height are positioned to fit each person. With the front part of the foot placed on the pedal (toe clips are helpful), the seat height is adjusted so that there is a slight bend of the knee when the pedal is in the down position (i.e., the legs are almost completely extended at the bottom of the downstroke). Patients are instructed to pedal 50 or 60 rpm. However, as previously stated, the pedalling frequency on an electromechanical cycle may vary without a significant change in power.[21]

Routine Procedure on Cycle or Treadmill

Routinely, a test is started with 2 minutes of rest, followed by 2 minutes of light exercise with the mouthpiece and nose clip snugly in place. If the patient is on the cycle, the 2 minute warm-up is done at "no load", also called free wheeling or unloaded pedalling. If on the treadmill, the warm-up is carried out at a slow belt speed (e.g., 2 mph) and zero elevation. The goal is to have the test completed in 10 to 12 minutes of incremental or ramp exercise, or in 6 minutes if the patient is elderly. The exercise may be (1) constant load, (2) incremental to maximal work rate (WRmax), or (3) ramp to WRmax.

Constant Load Exercise

A constant load is used if steady-state data are desired. The measurements are usually made at rest, during low-grade exercise, and during more stressful testing. Each test is performed for 4 to 6 minutes during which time a normal person will reach a "steady state" within 3 minutes. However, if the work rate is too high, the patient will NOT enter a steady state. Instead, the HR (heart rate), $\dot{V}_E$ (minute ventilation), and $\dot{V}O_2$ (minute oxygen consumption) will continue to rise. A useful measurement during constant-load exercise, either on the cycle or treadmill, is to subtract the $\dot{V}O_2$ at 3 minutes from the $\dot{V}O_2$ at 6 minutes ($\triangle \dot{V}O_2 6'-3'$). If the difference is zero (or a negative value) then steady-state conditions are present, and one is assured that the subject is exercising below the anaerobic threshold (AT). When the subject is above the AT, the 6'-3' value (ml's of O_2) is proportional to the increase in blood lactate (Figure 7).

Although constant load exercise (below the AT) requires several levels of work, it does permit estimation of the cardiac output (rebreathing techniques) and accurate measurement at different work rates, under steady-state conditions, of $\dot{V}_E$, $\dot{V}O_2$, $\dot{V}CO_2$, R, $\dot{V}_E/\dot{V}O_2$, $\dot{V}_E/\dot{V}CO_2$, HR, O_2/HR, BP, V_D/V_T, P(a-ET)CO_2, and P(A-a)O_2 (see DEFINITIONS p. 37). This information can be valuable to measure the patient's progress in rehabilitation programs and responses to therapy, such as the use of steroids in interstitial lung disease. The disadvantages of constant-load exercise are the increased time involved and tiring of the patient.

32

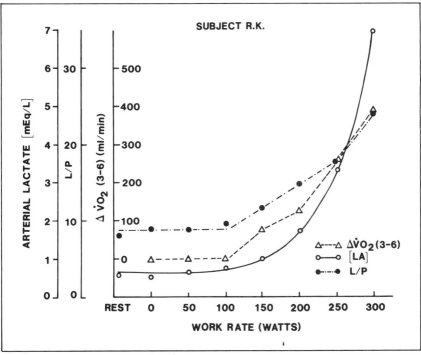

Figure 7. $\triangle \dot{V}O_2$(3-6), arterial lactate (LA), and lactate/pyruvate (L/P) at increasing work loads of exercise (constant loads) in a normal, well-trained subject. Note that for work below the AT (100 watts) the $\dot{V}O_2$(3-6) is zero. (*From* Whipp BJ, Wasserman K: Oxygen uptake kinetics for various intensities of constant-load work. J Appl Physiol 33: 351-356, 1972, with permission.)

Incremental Exercise

Following 2 minutes each of rest and warm-up, the patient performs incremental exercise, preferably on an electrically braked cycle ergometer. Usually the initial work rate is preselected at 20, 25, or 30 watts, depending upon the condition and daily activity of the patient. The level of exercise chosen is raised every minute by incrementing the same wattage until exhaustion or the test is stopped. For example, the subject starts a 1-minute incremental exercise test on the cycle at 25 watts while pedalling 60 rpm. Then the work rate is increased every minute as follows: 25 watts the first minute, 50 watts the second minute, 75 watts the third minute, 100 watts the fourth minute, etc., until the end of the test.

If incremental exercise is carried out on a treadmill, our routine, after rest and warm-up, is to raise the speed to as rapid a rate as the patient can handle comfortably at zero degrees elevation, e.g., walking level at 3.0 to 3.5 mph. After one minute, the work load is increased by raising the grade 3° every minute, but the speed is held constant. The end point again is exhaustion or ending the test.

Thus, using the 1-minute incremental exercise as described, maximal information can be obtained in a shorter period of time and with less tiring and faster recovery of the patient than employing several levels of steady-state exercise to exhaustion.

Ramp Exercise

Another method of cycle exercise is the **ramp** test which consists of **continuously** increasing the work rate to WRmax.[22,23] This protocol is accomplished with the aid of a computer which controls the work rate of the cycle. For each ramp slope (usually 20, 25 or 30 watts) the computer increments the signal once every second to the braking force of the flywheel of the cycle ergometer; e.g., for a ramp slope of 30 W min^{-1}, the work rate increment is 0.5 W each second. In this manner, the small incremental changes in work rate produce the same physiological changes that the subject would experience as if walking up a ramp. The major advantages of the ramp test are: (1) the production of a $\dot{V}O_2$ response which is linear; (2) the yield of a large amount of data in a short period of time with valid, reproducible parameters of aerobic function; (3) good acceptance by patients because of a smooth transition to higher work loads without a sudden, noticeable increase in pedal resistance.

Stopping the Exercise

Since the subject cannot talk while on the mouthpiece, a **signal code** needs to be prearranged for communication. For example, the patient may be instructed to point to the chest for angina, to the head for dizziness, or to the legs for claudication. Also when a patient is tiring greatly or wishes to stop for any reason, a convenient signal is to make a fist with the extended thumb pointed *downwards*. Conversely, the sign by the subject to continue the test is to make a fist with the extended thumb pointed *upwards*. Note that a slowing in the pedaling rate may be due to lack of attention or to fatigue.

The **goal of progressive exercise** (incremental or ramp) is for each subject to put forth his or her *best effort* to carry out the increasing work rate until further exercise becomes impossible. Ergo, most patients stop exercising because of exhaustion. However, there are a number of reasons why the patient or the supervising doctor may wish to stop the exercise.

Reasons to Stop the Test

(1) By the patient
  a. exhaustion
  b. dyspnea
  c. dizziness
  d. angina
  e. claudication
  f. pain in joints or tendons

(2) By the doctor
  a. EKG abnormalitiess[1]
     i. Ischemic changes: progressive ST-segment depression with horizontal or downslope of ST segment*, T wave inversion or the appearance of Q waves.
     ii. Rhythm disturbances: abnormally slow or rapid pulse, paroxysmal ventricular tachycardia, second or third degree heart block, onset of atrial fibrillation.
     iii. Appearance of a left bundle branch block (ST-segment index of ischemia is lost).

*If there is horizontal or downsloping ST-segment depression of 0.1 mv (1 mm) for at least 0.08 seconds after the "J" point, then 85% of these patients have significant coronary artery narrowing.[1]

  b. Blood pressure: *fall* in systolic BP more than 15-20 mmHg or a *rise* in excess of 250 mmHg. Diastolic BP in excess of 130 mmHg.
  c. Abnormally rapid respirations (e.g., >60/min)
  d. Palor, clamminess, or cyanosis
  f. Significant drop in SaO_2%. In our laboratory (elevation 800 ft/244 meters), exercise is discontinued if the oxygen saturation drops below 86%, which is equivalent to a PaO_2 of approximately 51-56 torr (pH = 7.3-7.4)
  g. **Note:** it is wise to limit some subjects to 85% of their maximal predicted heart rate (p. 39). This group includes the elderly and those patients with a history of heart disease. **Regarding ventricular ectopy:** The appearance of simple ventricular arrhythmias during exercise in healthy, asymptomatic persons is usually of **no** consequence. But in patients with **known** coronary artery disease, exercise induced ventricular arrhythmias may signal severe coronary artery disease or left ventricular dysfunction (Weiner DA, Levine SR: Primary Cardiology 12(3): 138-149, 1986).

Administration of Oxygen

Often, useful information can be gained by administering oxygen to hypoxemic patients while they are being exercised. The oxygen is given by nasal cannula at different flow rates, e.g., 1-5 L/min. The testing is done with the subject off the mouthpiece, and measurements are made using ear oximetry and (if indicated) arterial blood gases. When administering O_2 by nasal catheter it is not possible to measure the $\dot{V}O_2$ because of inherent inaccuracies, however, this measurement can be done with reasonable precision using a breath-by-breath analyzer and having the subject breathe an O_2 mixture (e.g., $F_IO_2 = 0.3, 0.4,$ or 0.5) from a large Douglas bag or meteorological balloon.

In our laboratory we routinely use low flow nasal O_2 on exercising patients who have significant O_2 desaturation (less than 90%) at rest or during exercise while breathing room air. Supplemental O_2 helps to relieve dyspnea, protects against cardiac arrhythmias and increases the rate of work performed.[24] **Frequently in patients with SEVERE COPD, the administration of O_2 permits exercise training when it otherwise would have been impossible!**

Post-Test Procedures

When the exercise test has been completed, the subjects are instructed to continue pedalling at "no load" for another 1-2 minutes before coming off the cycle. This maneuver prevents hypotension which is caused by pooling of blood in dilated vessels. High "R" values (> 1.2), due to hyperventilation, are common during the immediate post-exercise period. Monitoring of the blood pressure and EKG should continue for several minutes (usually 4-5 minutes) during the recovery period. Occasionally, ischemic changes appear on the electrocardiogram after completion of the test rather than during exercise. The heart should be examined for abnormal sounds.

CHAPTER 5
MATHEMATICAL POTPOURRI

Background information is necessary so that one can understand the basic physiologic principles involved in exercise testing. With this goal in mind, the present chapter includes definitions, predicted values, determinations, calculations and measurements.

Definitions

f_b(RR):   frequency of breathing (breaths/min)
V_T: tidal volume (BTPS; ml or L)
$\dot{V}_E$:   minute ventilation (BTPS; L/min)
V_T/FVC: ratio of tidal volume to forced vital capacity
V_D/V_T: ratio of dead space to tidal volume

$\dot{V}CO_2$:   carbon dioxide output (ml/min)
$\dot{V}O_2$:   oxygen uptake (ml/min)
R: respiratory exchange ratio $= \dot{V}CO_2/\dot{V}O_2 = $ RQ in the steady state
$\dot{V}O_2$/kg: oxygen uptake (ml/min) per kg of body weight
METS: $\dot{V}O_2$ (measured)/$\dot{V}O_2$ (resting); 1 MET $= 3.5$ ml O_2/kg/min, at rest

---

$\dot{V}_E/\dot{V}O_2$:   ventilatory equivalent for O_2; $\dot{V}_E$ is expressed as L/min, BTPS, and $\dot{V}O_2$ is expressed as L/min, STPD
$\dot{V}_E/\dot{V}CO_2$:   ventilatory equivalent for CO_2; the same units as for $\dot{V}_E/\dot{V}O_2$
$\dot{V}O_2/\dot{V}_E$:   true O_2 = ml of oxygen consumed (STPD) per liter of minute ventilation (BTPS).
$\dot{V}CO_2/\,\dot{V}_E$:   true CO_2 = ml of carbon dioxide produced (STPD) per liter of minute ventilation (BTPS).
HR (f_c):   heart rate = frequency of contractions (beats/min)
O_2/pulse: $\dot{V}O_2$/HR = oxygen uptake (ml/min) per heart beat
$P_{ET}O_2$:   tension of O_2 (end-tidal) in expired alveolar gas
$P_{ET}CO_2$:   tension of CO_2 (end-tidal) in expired alveolar gas
P(A-a)O_2:   alveolar-arterial O_2 tension difference
P(a-ET)CO_2:   arterial-end-tidal CO_2 tension difference

$SaO_2\%$:	arterial oxygen saturation expressed as percent

$\dot{V}_A$:	alveolar ventilation in an ideal lung to maintain $P_ACO_2 = PaCO_2$
$\dot{Q}$:	cardiac output or rate of blood flow through the lungs
$\dot{V}_A/Q$:	ratio of alveolar ventilation to pulmonary flood flow

ABG's:	arterial blood gases
pH:	$1/[H+] = 6.1 + \log[HCO_3^-/0.03 \times PaCO_2]$
PaO_2:	partial pressure of oxygen in arterial blood
$PaCO_2$:	partial pressure of carbon dioxide in arterial blood
HCO_3^-:	blood bicarbonate (mEq/L); calculated from the Henderson-Hasselbalch equation (see pH)

WR:	work rate; the absolute measure of the rate of doing work or the power output (force × distance per unit time), e.g., watts or kpm/min. Note: 1 watt = 6.12 kpm/min.
WRmax:	maximal work rate
WC:	work capacity = $\dot{V}O_2$max (subject)/predicted $\dot{V}O_2$max
AT:	anaerobic threshold; the highest O_2 consumption ($\dot{V}O_2$) during exercise above which a sustained arterial blood lactic acidosis occurs
BR:	breathing reserve = $1 - [\dot{V}_E max/MVV]$, where $\dot{V}_E max$ is the maximal minute ventilation (L/min, BTPS) and MVV is the maximal voluntary ventilation (L/min, BTPS)
HRR:	heart rate reserve = $1 - [(HRmax - HR\ rest)/(HR\ pred.max - HR\ rest)]$

ATPH:	gas volume at atmospheric temperature (°C), barometric pressure (P_B) and humidity ($P_{H_2O,t}$), where $P_{H_2O,t}$ = water vapor pressure at the temperature indicated.
ATPS:	gas volume at atmospheric temperature (°C), and barometric pressure (P_B) saturated with water vapor at the temperature indicated.
BTPS:	gas volume at body temperature (37°) and pressure (P_B), saturated with water vapor at 37°C (47 mmHg).
STPD:	gas volume at standard temperature (0°C), and barometric pressure (760 mmHg), dry.

Predicted Values for Human Performance

Before any exercise test is begun, the physician and the technician should know the **predicted maximal heart rate, oxygen uptake, minute ventilation and work rate.** A convenient practice is to write these four

38

maximal values on a blackboard in the exercise room where they can easily be seen. The determinations are as follows:

(1) Predicted maximal heart rate

Pred.HRmax = 220 − age (yrs). We use this calculation in preference to 210 − [0.65 × age (yrs)],[1.25] since the results more closely match the data published by the Tennessee Heart Association in 1972. The differences in HR between men and women are negligible.

(2) Predicted maximal oxygen uptake

FOR NORMAL AND OVERWEIGHT MALES, Hanson's (et al) modified values for cycle exercise of Bruce's treadmill calculations are:[25,26]

Normal Wt: Pred. $\dot{V}O_2$max (ml/min) = [50.72 − 0.372 age (yrs)] × Wt (kg);

Obese: Pred. $\dot{V}O_2$max (ml/min) = [50.72 − 0.372 age (yrs)] × [0.79 × Ht (cm) − 60.7].

FOR NORMAL AND OVERWEIGHT FEMALES, Wasserman's (et al) values are:[27]

Normal Wt: Pred. $\dot{V}O_2$max (ml/min) = [22.78 − 0.17 age (yrs)] × [42.8 + Wt (kg)];

Obese: Pred. $\dot{V}O_2$max (ml/min) = [14.81 − 0.11 age (yrs)] × Ht (cm).

Note: An individual can be classified as obese when the body mass index (BMI = weight [kg]/height [M^2]) is greater than 27.8 for men or 27.3 for women[28] (also, *Ann Intern Med* 103: 147-151, 1985).

FOR HEALTHY ADULTS, Shepard's, P. Astrand's, I. Astrand's, and Lange-Anderson's (et al) values are:[29-32]

Males: $\dot{V}O_2$max (L/min) = 4.2 − 0.032 age L/min (SD ± 0.4);
$\dot{V}O_2$max (ml/kg/min) = 60 − 0.55 age ml/kg/min (SD± 7.5)

Females: $\dot{V}O_2$max (L/min) = 2.6 − 0.014 age L/min (SD ± 0.4);
$\dot{V}O_2$max (ml/kg/min) = 48 − 0.37 age ml/kg/min (SD± 7.0)

Jones and Campbell use these values in their exercise laboratory.[1]

(3) Predicted maximal minute ventilation[1,33-35]

This value can be predicted by the following equation: MVV = FEV_1 × 35 or 40. Nevertheless, we continue to have the patient perform a 15-second maximal voluntary ventilation (15-sec MVV × 4 = 1-min MVV) and use this measured value rather than the calculated one. *Note that any significant difference between the "calculated" and "measured" MVV must be carefully investigated.* A poorly performed MVV may falsely make the subject appear to be "breathing limited".

39

(4) Predicted maximal work rate

The equation for predicting the WRmax is based on the fact that O_2 uptake in incremental or ramp exercise is linearly related to power and that O_2 uptake under basal conditions is approximatly 3.5 ml $O_2/kg/min$:

Pred. $\dot{V}O_2$max (ml/min) $= 2 \times$ kpm/min (@WRmax) $+$
[3.5 $\times$ Wt (kg)]; (1)[36]

rearranging,

Pred. WRmax (kpm/min) $= \dfrac{\text{pred.}\dot{V}O_2\text{max} - [3.5 \times \text{Wt (kg)}]}{2}$ (2)

expressed in watts,

Pred.WRmax (watts) $= \dfrac{\text{pred.}\dot{V}O_2\text{max} - [3.5 \times \text{Wt (kg)}]}{12.24}$ (3)

Notation: Equation No. 1 can be used in progressive exercise to see if O_2 uptake lies in a normal range in relationship to power. Likewise, under quasi-steady state conditions, the following equation by Wasserman[3] can be used to reasonably predict the $\dot{V}O_2$:

Pred.$\dot{V}O_2$ (ml/min) $= 5.8 \times$ Wt (kg) $+ 151 + [10.1 \times$ watts]; (4)
using kpm/min,
Pred.$\dot{V}O_2$ (ml/min) $= 5.8 \times$ Wt (kg) $+ 151 + [1.65 \times$ kpm/min]. (5)

Important Determinations from the Data

(1) Work capacity

To determine work capacity (WC), the subject's $\dot{V}O_2$max (maximal oxygen uptake) is measured to see how this value compares with the $\dot{V}O_2$max of a normal population of the same sex, age and size. Thus, WC $=$ subject's $\dot{V}O_2$max/pred.$\dot{V}O_2$max.

(2) Anaerobic threshold

As stated previously (p. 2), the anaerobic threshold (AT) is an important physiological event, defined by Wasserman and his colleagues as the highest $\dot{V}O_2$ during exercise above which a sustained lactic acidosis occurs.[2-5,7,37,38] As shown in Figure 8, the AT (also identified as θan) can be detected indirectly in progressive exercise by the simultaneous occurrence of these events:

(a) the $\dot{V}_E/\dot{V}O_2$ and $P_{ET}O_2$ systematically increase from their lowest values while the $\dot{V}_E/\dot{V}CO_2$ and the $P_{ET}CO_2$ remain virtually unchanged, resulting in "isocapnic buffering" for approximately 2 minutes;

(b) the R systematically rises from its nadir;

(c) the $\dot{V}_E$ and $\dot{V}CO_2$ increase linearly up to the AT, at which point they become non-linear to the $\dot{V}O_2$ by rising more steeply. If there is any discrepancy between the preceding values, the $\dot{V}_E/\dot{V}O_2$ is felt to be the most reliable.

Note: If the AT is "indeterminate" (an occasional event), then the examiner has three reasonable options: (1) Simply state on the exercise report that the AT cannot be determined; (2) Repeat the exercise test another day using a different work load; e.g., try increasing the work rate by 5 watts/min. We have noted that if the work rate is too low, the subject may slowly "pass through" the AT without having a sharp nadir; (3) Use **constant load** exercise to determine the AT. This maneuver is time-consuming (because of repeated tests) but is effective. The AT will be just prior to the work rate where a significant difference begins to appear between the $\dot{V}O_2$ at 3 minutes and at 6 minutes.

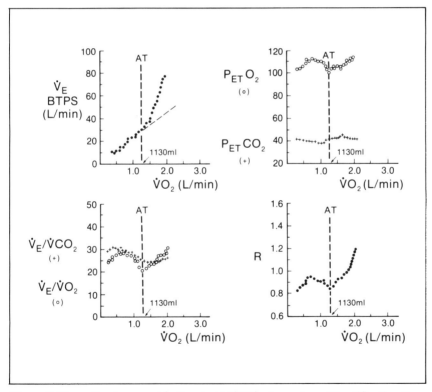

Figure 8. The author's anaerobic threshold (AT) is shown here. Identification lines have been drawn for each panel, marking the AT at the nadirs of the $\dot{V}_E/\dot{V}O_2$, $P_{ET}O_2$ and R. Note leveling of the $P_{ET}CO_2$ and $\dot{V}_E/\dot{V}CO_2$ at the AT; also non-linearity of the $\dot{V}_E$ at the AT.

41

(3) Breathing reserve

The breathing reserve (BR) represents the unused fraction of maximal voluntary ventilation: $BR = 1 - [\dot{V}_E max/MVV]$, where $\dot{V}_E max$ is the ventilation at maximal exercise and the MVV is the maximal voluntary ventilation at rest.[39]

(4) Heart rate reserve

The heart rate reserve (HRR) represents the unused fraction of the heart rate at maximal work levels.[39] Taking into account the subject's resting heart rate, the final equation is:

$$HRR = 1 - [(HRmax - HRrest)/(HRpred.max - HRrest)].$$

(5) Oxygen-pulse[1]

This useful bit of information is obtained simply by dividing the subject's $\dot{V}O_2$ by the pulse, thus yielding the ml's of oxygen consumed per heart beat at a given work load. O_2/pulse (also termed O_2/HR) is related to stroke volume (SV) as shown by the following equations:

Whereas $\dot{Q} = \dot{V}O_2/C(a-\bar{v})O_2$, and $\dot{Q} = SV \times HR$,

then $\dot{V}O_2/C(a-\bar{v})O_2 = SV \times HR$.

Rearranging, $\dot{V}O_2/HR = SV \times C(a-\bar{v})O_2$.

(6) Dead space — tidal volume ratio[40]

The ratio of physiological dead space to tidal volume measures wasted ventilation and can be calculated using Enghoff's modification of the Bohr equation: $V_D/V_T = (PaCO_2 - P_ECO_2)/PaCO_2$. An arterial blood gas sample is drawn to obtain the $PaCO_2$ value, and the partial pressure of mixed expired CO_2 is determined from the equation: $P_ECO_2 = (\dot{V}CO_2/[\dot{V}_E-\dot{V}_D valve \times fb]) \times 0.863$. The V_D/V_T also can be readily calculated by a different method. Since the V_T values appear in the computer print-out data, V_D can be determined by subtracting alveolar ventilation ($\dot{V}_A$) from minute ventilation ($\dot{V}_E$) in the following manner:

$V_D = [(\dot{V}_E-\dot{V}_A)/f_b]$-valve V_D, where $\dot{V}_A = (\dot{V}CO_2/PaCO_2) \times 0.863$, and valve V_D = valve dead space.

Note: some exercise physiologists do not subtract the valve dead space, however, this issue has not been settled.

(7) Alveolar-arterial PO_2 difference

In calculating $P(A-a)O_2$, the value for PaO_2 is obtained from the arterial blood gas sample, and the partial pressure of O_2 in the alveolus is determined as follows:

$$P_AO_2 \text{ (room air)} = [(PB - 47) \times 0.2093] - [PaCO_2 \times (0.2093 + \frac{0.7907}{R})].$$

A dynamic factor in this equation is "R" ($\dot{V}CO_2/\dot{V}O_2$) which changes throughout exercise, however, *at rest* many laboratories simply assume that the subject's R is normal (approximately 0.80) and therefore, $PaCO_2$ is multiplied by 1.2 or 1.25.

(8) Arterial-end-tidal PCO_2 difference

In calculating $P(a\text{-}ET)CO_2$ difference, the value for $PaCO_2$ is obtained from the arterial blood gas sample. To derive the partial pressure of CO_2 in the end-tidal expired air ($P_{ET}CO_2$), gas samples are taken at the mouth and measured by the gas analyzer as % (fraction of CO_2). The computer then converts the % of CO_2 into partial pressure using the following equation:

$$P_{ET}CO_2 = F_{ET}CO_2 \times (P_B - P_{H2O,t}), \text{ e.g.,}$$
$$P_{ET}CO_2 = 0.05 \times (750 - 32) = 36 \text{ torr.}$$

(9) "R" and the respiratory quotient[37]

The respiratory quotient (RQ) is the gas exchange ratio at the lungs *in a steady state*. Since conditions always change rapidly in incremental or ramp exercise, a more appropriate term to use here is "R". The R value ($\dot{V}CO_2/\dot{V}O_2$) is a useful indicator to follow. When R rises above 1.0 in progressive exercise, usually the subject must stop within 2-3 minutes because of increasing lactic acidosis; and when the R crosses 1.1 the subject generally is within one minute of being unable to continue. R at $\dot{V}O_2$max is 1.2 ± 0.12. The highest R values (1.59 ± 0.19) are found following exercise in the first two minutes of recovery. Marked hyperventilation is noted during this period.

Other Calculations and Measurements

(1) Oxygen uptake:[1]
$$\dot{V}O_2 \text{ (ml/min, STPD)} = [V_I STPD \times 0.2093) - (V_E STPD \times F_EO_2)] \times 10^3;$$

rearranging, $\dot{V}O_2$ (STPD) $= [(0.2093 \times \dfrac{1-F_EO_2-F_ECO_2}{0.7904}) - F_EO_2] \times V_E$ (STPD) x 10^3.

(2) Carbon dioxide output:[1]
$$\dot{V}CO_2 \text{ (ml/min, STPD)} = F_ECO_2 \times \dot{V}_E \text{ (STPD)} \times 10^3.$$

(3) Standardization of gas volumes for temperature and pressure:[41]

When the pneumotachometer is located in the *inspiratory* line, then

$$\dot{V}_E \text{ (BTPS)} = \dot{V}_I \text{ (ATPH)} \times [273 + 37/273 + t] \times$$
$$[P_B - P_{H2O,t}/P_B - 47],$$

where $P_{H_2O,t}$ is the pressure exerted by partially saturated water vaper at room temperature (t). When the pneumotachometer is located in the *expiratory* line, then the same equation above also applies for calculating $\dot{V}_E$ except that $P_{H_2O,t}$ = fully saturated aqueous vapor pressure at room temperature.

To convert gas volumes from BTPS to STPD, the following equation is used:

$\dot{V}E$ (STPD) = $\dot{V}_E$ (BTPS) × [273/273 + 37] × [PB − 47/760].

To convert gas volumes from ATPH to STPD the following equation is used:

$\dot{V}_E$ (STPD) = $\dot{V}_E$ (ATPH) × [273/273 + t] × [P_B − $P_{H_2O,t}$/760].

(4) The Haldane transformation:[42]

There is a slight difference in the volume of inspired and expired air except when R = 1.0, i.e., when $\dot{V}CO_2$ = $\dot{V}O_2$. Thus, if the pneumotachometer is in the *inspiratory* line, the Haldane correction to calculate $\dot{V}_E$ is carried out in the following manner:

$\dot{V}_E$ (STPD) = $\dot{V}_I$ (STPD) × F_IN_2/F_EN_2, where F_IN_2 = 0.7904 and F_EN_2 = (1 − F_EO_2 − F_ECO_2), dry.

If the pneumotachometer is on the *expiratory* side then $\dot{V}_I$ is calculated as follows:

$\dot{V}_I$ (STPD) = $\dot{V}_E$ (STPD) × F_EN_2/0.7904, dry.

(5) Humidity

Humidity is the bane of the physiologist since the concentration of any gas is affected by the presence of water vapor. The relative humidity of ambient air can be measured by a hygrometer (Digital Hygrometer-Thermometer, made by Fisher Scientific). If this instrument is not available, one can utilize the O_2 analyzer (which has been standardized using dry O_2) by taking a reading of % O_2 in the room air without drying the sample. The concentration of the "wet" O_2 obtained (e.g., 20.7%) is entered into the following equation to calculate atmostpheric water pressure in mmHg:

$$\frac{\% \text{ dry } O_2 - \% \text{ wet } O_2}{\% \text{ dry } O_2} \times P_B = P_{H_2O,t} \quad (1)$$

$$\frac{20.93 - 20.7}{20.93} \times 747 = P_{H_2O,t} \quad (2)$$

$$0.010989 \times 747 = 8.2 \text{ mmHg.} \quad (3)$$

If the room temperature is 21°C ($P_{H_2O,21°C}$ [saturated] = 18.7 mmHg), then the relative humidity is: 8.2 ÷ 18.7 = 44%.

44

CHAPTER 6
INTERPRETATION OF EXERCISE RESULTS

Step-By-Step Program

Exercise testing is a chain of events with the optimum results being no better than the "weakest link in the chain." The interpretation of large amounts of data obtained by modern, computerized equipment can be an unpleasant experience to the innovate. Nevertheless, once having gained adequate basic knowledge, the evaluation of dynamic, physiologic data can be exciting and rewarding. The approach used here is rather pragmatic, i.e., to take one step at a time in converting the data into a meaningful report.

1. Is the exercise maximal or submaximal?

Good effort and patient cooperation are required to achieve maximal exercise! The degree of exercise can be determined by observing the following criteria at WRmax: (a) a blood bicarbonate below 21 mEq/L is synonymous with good effort; (b) a drop of 4 mEq or more in the HCO_3^- (as compared to the value at rest) indicates that lactic acid production has been sufficient enough to constitute the exercise as being "maximal". The values for HCO_3^- are obtained from the blood gas samples drawn pre-exercise (at rest) and near the end of exercise. These bicarbonate values are not measured directly but are determined indirectly from the Henderson-Hasselbalch equation:

$$pH = 6.1 + LOG \frac{HCO_3^-}{0.03 \times PaCO_2}.$$

Additional supportive evidence of a maximal exercise are an R value above 1.09 and a significant drop in the pH.

2. What is the subject's work capacity?[3]

The work capacity (WC) is normal when the subject's $\dot{V}O_2max$ is 90-100% of his or her *predicted* $\dot{V}O_2max$ (p.). Borderline = 85-90%, and reduced = 84% or less. If the work capacity is normal, then the anaerobic threshold is uniformly normal (there may be rare exceptions). Under these circumstances (normal WC) the subject may be normal, obese, or have mild heart or mild lung disease. If the WC is *low,* then the AT (anaerobic threshold) becomes a *critical point* for differentiating circulatory

45

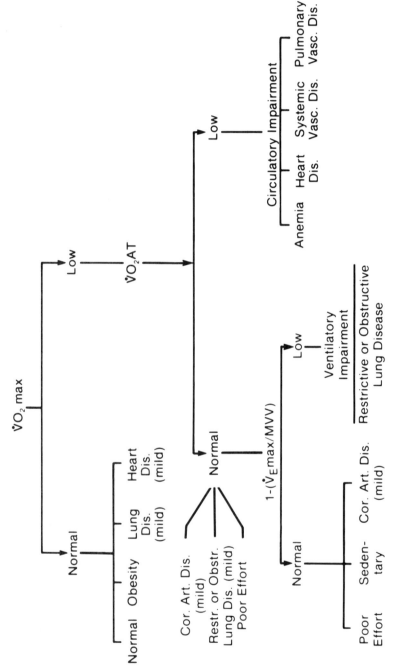

Figure 9. Wasserman's flow chart is especially helpful in the differential diagnosis of dyspnea. The vital relationship of the anaerobic threshold is clearly seen in this schema. The $\dot{V}O_2AT$ is **low** if less than 40% of the subject's predicted $\dot{V}O_2$max and indicates circulatory impairment. The breathing reserve is **low** if $1-(\dot{V}_Emax/MVV)$ is less than 30%. (Adapted *from* Wasserman K: The anaerobic threshold measurement in exercise testing. *Clinics In Chest Medicine,* 5(1): 77-88, 1984; with permission.)

impairment from a variety of conditions as shown in Wasserman's diagnostic flow chart in Figure 9.

3. What is the subject's anaerobic threshold?[3-7]

An extremely useful determinant is to divide the subject's $\dot{V}O_2$ at the anaerobic threshold by the predicted $\dot{V}O_2$max ($\dot{V}O_2$AT/pred. $\dot{V}O_2$max). Normal = 40% or higher and low = 39% or less.[7] A low $\dot{V}O_2$AT indicates circulatory impairment involving the heart, pulmonary circulation, systemic circulation, or peripheral vascular system (Figure 9); anemia also must be ruled out. A normal $\dot{V}O_2$AT in the presence of a low work capacity may be due to a number of factors: poor patient effort; an exceptionally sedentary life style (poor fitness or state of being deconditioned); mild coronary artery disease or ventilatory impairment secondary to obstructive, or restrictive lung disease. The heart rate at the anaerobic threshold (HR-AT) is another important value which is useful in disability evaluations, rehabilitation programs, and writing exercise prescriptions (Chapter 10).

4. What is the subject's respiratory status?[25,39]

Ventilatory limitation is implied when the breathing reserve (BR) is less than 30% of the subject's MVV or when the MVV-$\dot{V}_E$max is 15 liters or less. Uniformly, the BR is normal when the work capacity is normal. One should keep in mind, however, that a well-motivated athlete or well-conditioned individual may have a BR that is less than 0.30 at WRmax. In healthy persons, the respiratory rate (f_b) rarely approaches 60 breaths per minute; V_T never exceeds the individual's inspiratory capacity (IC), and the highest V_T/FVC ratio possible is in the range of 0.55 to 0.60. In restrictive lung disease, the V_T fails to increase normally as the work rate increases; thus, to meet the ventilatory demands of exercise, f_b may significantly exceed 60 breaths per minute ($V_T \times f_b = V_E$).

5. What is the subject's cardiac status?[1,3,25,39,43]

Cardiac status is determined by:
(a) the rate, rhythm, and configuration of the electrocardiogram (p. 35);
(b) the response of the subject's blood pressure to increasing work rates:
   i. failure of the systolic pressure to rise (indicates left ventricular dysfunction);
   ii. hypertensive response, systolic or diastolic.
(c) the heart rate reserve (HRR) as defined on page 42;
(d) the O_2/pulse.

Normally, a low HRR at WRmax equates with a good effort and maximal work. In disease states, however, the HRR may be disproportionately low when compared to the level of work being performed; e.g., the presence of a low HRR (rapid pulse) during mild exercise. A high

HRR (slow pulse) may be due to poor effort, conduction disease, beta blockage from drugs, or the fact that the subject is a superbly trained athlete. A high HRR also is seen in patients with a breathing impairment which is severe enough to limit exercise and thus limit their heart rate (HR).

Regarding the O_2/pulse ($\dot{V}O_2$/HR), the approximate value at WRmax for this important determinant is 8.0 ml/heart beat or higher for *adult females* and 12 ml/beat or higher for *adult males* (exceptions may occur in small or older persons who have a low $\dot{V}O_2$max). A more exact value can be calculated by dividing the subject's predicted $\dot{V}O_2$max by his or her predicted HRmax. Lower values at maximal work rates or a leveling or fall in the O_2/pulse during progressive exercise indicate cardiac impairment. As shown in the equation on page 42, O_2/pulse is the product of stroke volume (SV) and the arteriovenous O_2 content difference [C(a-v̄)O_2]. Causes of a low O_2/pulse are: (1) poor motivation; (2) musculoskeletal limitation; (3) ventilatory limitation. Sue and Hansen (*Clinics in Chest Medicine,* 5(1): 89-98, 1984) pointed out that if factors 1-3 can be excluded, then a low O_2/pulse may be predictive of cardiovascular limitation.

6. What is the subject's pulmonary gas exchange status?[25,40,44-48]

The relationship of ventilation to perfusion ($\dot{V}/\dot{Q}$) is determined by three factors, all of which are indices of pulmonary gas exchange:

(a) V_D/V_T: In normal subjects at rest the V_D/V_T is approximately 0.30 to 0.35 and falls below 0.25 during maximal exercise. At WRmax, a V_D/V_T value above 0.25 in younger subjects and above 0.30 in older subjects represents a mismatching of ventilation and perfusion (dead space ventilation) which may be seen in rapid, shallow breathing, chronic obstructive lung disease, or pulmonary vascular occlusion.[25,30,38]

(b) P(A-a)O_2: In subjects with normal ventilation/perfusion ratios, the alveolar-arterial PO_2 difference is below 21 torr on room air while at rest. During vigorous exercise, some widening of the PO_2 difference may normally occur.[3] In elderly patients, a P(A-a)O_2 higher than 34 torr or a PaO_2 below 75 torr should be considered as abnormal during heavy exercise above the AT (anaerobic threshold) at WRmax.[25] In younger patients, however, a normal response during maximal exercise is a PO_2 difference less than 21 torr and a PaO_2 which is at least 80 torr or higher with a mean of 90 torr.

(c) P(a-ET)CO_2: Normally this useful value is slightly positive at rest (approximately $+2.5$ torr) and becomes negative (approximately -4.0 torr) during exercise.[3,25] A positive value during heavy exercise indicates impaired gas exchange (ventilation but no perfusion) and may be seen in chronic obstructive lung disease, restrictive lung disease, and pulmonary vascular disease. Often an abnormal a-ET CO_2 difference is accompanied by hypoxemia, an increased A-a O_2 difference and a high V_D/V_T.

CHAPTER 7
WRITING THE REPORT

Modern, computerized equipment and competent technical help are important factors in obtaining reliable results from cycle or treadmill testing. Once the results are obtained, however, the physician in charge of the exercise test is responsible for proper interpretation of the data and for writing the report. It is common knowledge that there is "no such thing" as an emergency exercise test; nevertheless, the information gained by carrying out stress testing on thoughtfully selected patients can have far reaching implications in the management of these individuals.

To achieve this goal, namely **writing the report,** a checklist in outline form is provided below to assess the patient's metabolic, cardiopulmonary, and gas exchange dynamics. This outline can be easily transformed into an integrated report form, like the one used here at the University of Iowa Hospitals and Clinics (Figure 10). In addition, Wasserman's diagnostic flow chart (Figure 9) is helpful, from a physiological standpoint, in categorizing the patient's fitness or impairment.

Guidelines for Writing the Report

1. **Pre-exercise information**
   a. Reason for the test.
   b. History (occupation, life style, habits, diet, medications, symptoms, past history, etc.).
   c. Physical examination (ht., wt., pulse, temp., BP, exam of chest, and heart, etc.).
   d. Laboratory data (CBC, UA, PFT's, ABG's, EKG, CXR).
   e. Clinical diagnosis.

2. **Type of test performed**
   a. Cycle ergometer: incremental or ramp; watts/min or kpm/min (1.0 watt = 6.12 kpm).
   b. Treadmill: speed, elevation, time intervals.

UNIVERSITY OF IOWA HOSPITALS & CLINICS   NAME:
CARDIOPULMONARY EXERCISE LABORATORY   AGE: SEX: HT: WT:
    HOSPITAL NO:
    DATE: REF.MD:

HISTORY:

Predicted Values

PFT's: $\dot{V}O_2$max _____
    HRmax _____

EXERCISE TEST: O_2/HR _____
    WRmax _____

     pH PO_2 PCO_2 HCO_3 "R"

Rest: MVV

WRmax:

		NORMAL	PATIENT
GEN-ERAL	WORK CAPACITY: $\dot{V}O_2$max/pred. $\dot{V}O_2$max	>85%	
	ANAEROBIC THRESHOLD: $\dot{V}O_2$AT/pred. $\dot{V}O_2$max	>40%	
RESPIR-ATORY	BREATHING RESERVE: $1-(\dot{V}_E$max/MVV); also MVV $-\dot{V}_E$max . .	>30% ; >15 L	
	f_b: Rest → WRmax	8 → 60/min	
	V_T/FVC: Rest → WRmax	0.15 → 0.60	
$\dot{V}/\dot{Q}$	P(A-a)O_2: Rest → WRmax		
	V_D/V_T: Rest → WRmax	0.35 → <0.25	
	P(a-ET)CO_2: Rest → WRmax	+2 → <0	
CAR-DIAC	HR RESERVE: 1-[(HRmax-HRrest)/(HRpred.max-HRrest)] . .		
	HR-AT: (heart beat @ AT)		
	O_2/Pulse: Rest → WRmax		
	BLOOD PRESSURE:		
	EKG:		

REASON EXERCISE STOPPED:

INTERPRETATION:

Copyright: 1985, D.C. ZAVALA, M.D.   SIGNATURE _____

Figure 10.

50

3. **State subject's response**
   a. Work rate that exercise was terminated.
   b. Degree of cooperation.
   c. Effort made.
   d. Any significant symptoms, e.g., chest pain, dizziness, claudication.

4. **Determine if maximal or submaximal exercise**
   a. If maximal,
      (1) "R" ($\dot{V}CO_2/\dot{V}O_2$) rises over 1.09
      (2) HCO_3^- drops 4 mEq or more.
      (3) pH usually falls significantly.
   b. If submaximal,
      (1) none of the above occur.

5. **Calculate work capacity (WC) @ WRmax**

   $$\%WC = \frac{\dot{V}O_2max}{pred. \ \dot{V}O_2max}$$

   Comments:
   Normal = 90% or higher.
   Borderline = 85-89%.
   Low = 84% or less (indicates unfitness, poor effort or disease state).

6. **Determine ratio of $\dot{V}O_2$ at the anaerobic threshold to predicted $\dot{V}O_2max$**

   $$\% = \frac{\dot{V}O_2AT}{pred. \ \dot{V}O_2max}$$

   Comments:
   Normal = 40% or higher. In addition to the $\dot{V}O_2AT$, note the HR-AT and the $\dot{V}_EAT$.
   Low = 39% or less. A low AT indicates circulatory impairment.

7. **Determine pulmonary status @ WRmax**
   a. $V_T \times f_b = \dot{V}_E$
   Comments:
   Normal = the respiratory rate is less than 60/min; the V_T reaches 55-60% of the vital capacity at WRmax and never exceeds the IC.
   Restrictive lung disease = characterized by early limitation of V_T with the increase in $\dot{V}_E$ being achieved by a high f_b.

b. MVV $- \dot{V}_E =$ _____ liters

Comments:
Abnormal = 15 liters or less.

c. Breathing reserve (BR)

$$\%BR = 1 - [\frac{\dot{V}_E max}{MVV}]$$

Comments:
Normal = there is no breathing limitation at maximal exercise.
Abnormal = less than 30%, which indicates a breathing limitation.
Exceptions are well motivated athletes.

8. Determine cardiac status @ WRmax

a. Electrocardiogram.

Comments:
Check for rhythm disturbances, ST-T changes, Q waves, enlarged
P waves, etc.

b. Blood pressure.

Comments:
Stop exercise if systolic BP falls or if it rises over 250 mmHg.

c. O_2/pulse ($\dot{V}O_2$/HR)

Comments:
Results are invalid when patient is on a beta-adrenergic blocker.
Approximate normal = 8 ml O_2/beat or higher for adult females
and 12 ml O_2/beat or higher for adult males; exceptions are small,
older persons. To calculate a more exact value, divide the
predicted $\dot{V}O_2$ max by the predicted HRmax.
Abnormal = lower values than above; also a plateau or fall during
progressive exercise.

d. HR reserve (HRR)

$$HRR = 1 - [\frac{HRmax - HR\ rest}{HR\ pred.\ max - HR\ rest}]$$

Comments:
Results are invalid when patient is on beta blockers.
Normal = small HRR at WRmax. (There is a cardiac limit at
maximal exercise)
Abnormal = small HRR early in exercise.

9. Determine gas exchange ($\dot{V}/\dot{Q}$) @ rest and WRmax

a. V_D/V_T

Comments:
Normal = 0.3-0.35 at rest $\rightarrow$ <0.25 at WRmax. Exceptions are
elderly persons whose value should be less than 0.30 at WRmax.

Abnormal = rise during exercise or failure to fall below values shown above at WRmax.

b. $P(A-a)O_2$

Comments:
Normal = less than 21 torr during rest or stress testing although some widening may occur during heavy exercise. Exceptions are elderly persons whose upper normal limit is 34 torr at WRmax.

c. $P(a-ET)CO_2$

Comments:
Normal = +2.5 torr at rest with a fall below zero at WRmax. Usual range is +2.5 torr at rest to −4.0 torr at WRmax.
Abnormal = a value above zero torr at WRmax.

10. **State reason for stopping exercise (see pages 34, 35.)**
   a. By the subject
   b. By the physician

11. **Perform post-exercise follow-up**
   a. Electrocardiogram
   Comments:
   Occasionally, abnormal ST-T changes occur *after* the test.
   b. Blood pressure
   Comments:
   BP response during recovery phase is important; see how long it takes for the BP to return to pre-exercise levels.
   c. Exam of chest and heart
   Comments:
   Check the chest for wheezing, rales, etc. **Examine the heart** for murmurs or unusual sounds.

12. **Review exercise data**
   This your job. Make sure that all calculations are correct.

13. **Complete the report form** (See Figure 10.)

14. **Make recommendations**
   Comments:
   When appropriate: referral, exercise prescription, disability report, rehabilitation evaluation, additional lab studies, etc.

CHAPTER 8
CASE REPORT WITH STEP-BY-STEP INTERPRETATION

The following case report was selected from our patient's files to illustrate the value of exercise testing in **differentiating cardiac from respiratory limitation.** The report is done in step-by-step fashion to re-emphasize the points made in Chapter 6 (Interpretation of Exercise Results) and Chapter 7 (Writing the Report).

Case Report (See Exhibit 3 in Chapter 9)

The patient is a physically active young woman, age 19 years old, who was seen in the medical clinic at the University of Iowa Hospitals and Clinics. She presented with a chief complaint of shortness of breath and lightheadedness which occurred only during considerable exertion at ballet practice and never during light exercise. She gave no past history of asthma or wheezing. Physical examination revealed a healthy appearing individual:

Ht. 170 cm (67 inches),
Wt. 58.6 kg (129 lbs.),
Pulse 67/min,
BP 102/84 mmHg,
Temp 37°C (98.6°F)

The chest was clear to percussion and auscultation, and the heart tones were normal. No cardiac murmurs or unusual heart sounds were heard. The remainder of the examination was normal. Laboratory data: A complete blood count and urinalysis were normal. Pulmonary function tests revealed the FVC to be 3.82 L (87%), FEV_1 3.5 L (99%), FEV_1/FVC 92%, MVV 101 L (80%), and DLco 94%. Resting arterial blood gas values showed the pH to be 7.42, PO_2 94 torr, PCO_2 38 torr, HCO_3^- 25 mEq, and $P(A-a)O_2$ 7 torr. An electrocardiogram and chest roentgenogram were also normal. The clinical diagnosis was deferred, and an exercise test was ordered. The interpretation of the test results is shown below, item by item, as outlined in Chapter 7. **The raw data on the computer printout is**

NAME: K.M. DATE: 1-27-84 Hosp. No. _____ U. of Iowa Hospitals and Clinics

SEX: F AGE: 19 yrs.

BSA: 1.68 sqm
WT: 129 LB, 58.6 KG
HT: 67 in., 170 cm

EXERCISE MODE: RAMP 25 WATTS/min

SMOKING HISTORY: NONE

CLINICAL INFORMATION: DYSPNEA, DIZZINESS ON EXERTION
INTERVAL LENGTH: 60 seconds

ENVIRONMENT: PB (torr): 749 TEMP (C): 22 HUMIDITY (%): 14

MAXIMAL EXERCISE VALUES:

		PREDICTED	ACTUAL	% OF PREDICTED
V_E max	(L/min)	BTPS: 123	54	44
	(L/min)	STPD: 97		
VO2 max	(ml/min)	STPD: 1982	1850	93
	(ml/kg/min)	STPD: 35		
HR max	(beats/min)	: 201	169	84
O2 PULSE	(ml/beat)	STPD: 9.9	11	100+
RATE PRESSURE PRODUCT		: 350 ± 44	210	60

STATIC PFT VALUES:

	PREDICTED	ACTUAL	% OF PREDICTED
FVC	4.40	3.82	87
FEV1	3.56	3.50	99
FEV1/FVC	0.81	0.92	
FEF 25-75	4.00	4.68	117
PEF	6.88	7.35	107
MVV	125	101	80

Table 1

55

NAME: K.M. DATE: 1-27-84 Hosp. No. _____ U. of Iowa Hospitals and Clinics

60 sec INTERVAL	1	2	3	4	5	6
Power (watts)	Rest	Rest	No Load	No Load	0-25 W	25-50 W
VE BTPS (L/min)	12.7	10.5	17	15.5	15	17.5
Resp Rate (br/min)	18	19	19	18	17	19
VT BTPS (ml)	701	553	971	871	883	934
VT/VC (fract.)	0.18	0.14	0.25	0.23	0.23	0.25
VD/VT (fract.)	0.32					
VO2 (ml/min)	412	316	594	520	491	605
VO2 (ml/kg/min)	7	5.4	10	8.9	8.4	10
Mets	2	1.5	2.9	2.5	2.4	2.9
VCO2 (ml/min)	327	263	504	456	440	522
R	0.794	0.847	0.85	0.876	0.895	0.864
VE/VCO2	39	39	34	34	34	34
VE/VO2	31	33	29	30	30	29
PETCO2 (mmHg)	36.5	37	36.4	36.3	37.3	36.4
PETO2 (mmHg)	96.9	99.3	97.5	101	97.8	100
Heart Rate (bpm)	63	67	85	81	82	87
O2 Pulse (ml/beat)	6.5	4.7	7	6.4	6	6.9
Systolic BP (mmHg)	102		110		112	114
Diastolic BP (mmHg)	84		84		84	84
Ear Oxim O2 Sat (%)	97.5	97	97.1	97.6	97.4	97.7
PO2 (mmHg)	94					
PCO2 (mmHg)	38					
pH	7.42					
BICARB (mEq/L)	25					
P(A-a)O2 (mmHg)	7					
P(a-ET)CO2 (mmHg)	+1.5					

Table 1 (cont.)

Table 1 (cont.)

NAME: K.M.	DATE: 1-27-84		Hosp. No.___		U. of Iowa Hospitals and Clinics
60 sec INTERVAL	7	8	9	10	11
Power (watts)	50-75 W	75-100 W	100-125 W	125-150 W	150-175 W
VE BTPS (L/min)	18.2	25.1	32.4	46.7	54.2
Resp Rate (br/min)	18	22	24	27	30
VT BTPS (ml)	1050	1140	1350	1730	1807
VT/VC (fract.)	0.27	0.30	0.35	0.45	0.47
VD/VT (fract.)					0.16
VO2 (ml/min)	832	1150	1400	1670	1850
VO2 (ml/kg/min)	14	20	24	29	32
Mets	4.1	5.6	6.8	8.1	9
VCO2 (ml/min)	617	973	1230	1810	2140
R	0.741	0.85	0.881	1.08	1.16
VE/VCO2	29	26	26	26	25
VE/VO2	22	21	23	28	29
PETCO2 (mmHg)	39.1	40.5	42.6	42.3	42.9
PETO2 (mmHg)	91.8	92.2	94.9	102	104
Heart Rate (bpm)	99	109	127	156	169
O2 Pulse (ml/beat)	8.4	11	11	11	11
Systolic BP (mmHg)	120	124	124	126	124
Diastolic BP (mmHg)	84	84	84	84	84
Ear Oxim O2 Sat (%)	97	96.8	96.6	96.7	97
PO2 (mmHg)					99
PCO2 (mmHg)					43
pH					7.30
BICARB (mEq/L)					21
P(A-a)O2 (mmHg)					10
P(a-ET)CO2 (mmHg)					0

shown in Table 1 (p.p. 55-57).

Item 1.

The pre-exercise information is given above.

Item 2.

An exercise test was carried out on a cycle ergometer using a breath-by-breath analyzer (MGC Exercise System 2000) with a ramp slope of 25 watts·min^{-1}.

Item 3.

The *patient was cooperative* and made a good effort. The exercise was terminated by the physician (and patient) upon completing 150-175 watts. She experienced shortness of breath and dizziness during the last 2-3 minutes of exercise.

Item 4.

The *exercise was maximal* as evidenced by a drop in the bicarbonate of 4 mEq (from 25 to 21 mEq), an "R" at WRmax of 1.16, and a drop in pH from 7.42 at rest to 7.30 at WRmax.

Item 5.

The *work capacity* at WRmax was normal:
WC $=$ 1850 ml O_2/1982 ml O_2 $=$ 93%.

Item 6.

The *anaerobic threshold* was normal (Figures 11,12):
1150 ml O_2/1982 ml O_2 $=$ 58%.

At the anaerobic threshold the subject's work rate (WR-AT) was at a ramp slope of 75-100 watts, the HR (HR-AT) was 109 beats/min, the $\dot{V}_E$ ($\dot{V}_E$AT) was 25.1 L/min, the "R" (R-AT) was 0.85 and the $\dot{V}O_2$ ($\dot{V}O_2$AT) was 1150 ml/min.

Item 7.

The *ventilatory response* at WRmax was normal:
a. V_T (1807 ml) $\times$ f_b (30/min) $=$ $\dot{V}_E$ (54.2 L/min);
  V_T (1807 ml) / FVC (3.82 L) $=$ 47%.
b. MVV (101 L/min) $-$ $\dot{V}_E$ (54.2 L/min) $=$ 46.8 L.
c. BR $= 1 - [\dfrac{\dot{V}_E \ (54.2 \ L)}{MVV \ (101 \ L)}] = 46\%$ (ample breathing reserve).

Item 8.

The *cardiac response* was abnormal:
a. The EKG showed mildly prominent P waves at work rates above 100 watts.

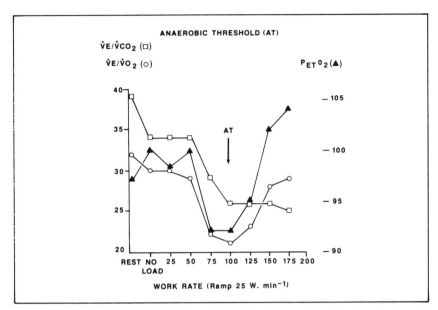

Figure 11. **Case 3:** The anaerobic threshold (AT) is clearly identified (arrow) in this patient at the nadirs of the $\dot{V}_E/\dot{V}O_2$ and $P_{ET}O_2$ (100 watts) at which time the $\dot{V}_E/\dot{V}CO_2$ is virtually unchanged.

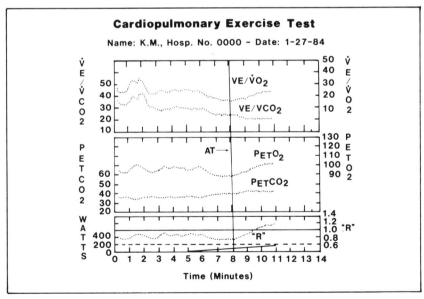

Figure 12. **Case 3:** Computer printout in graphic form of the significant exercise data ($\dot{V}_E/\dot{V}O_2$, $\dot{V}_E/\dot{V}CO_2$, $P_{ET}O_2$, $P_{ET}CO_2$) used to identify the anaerobic threshold (AT). A "cursor" appears on the CRT screen which is positioned by the operator to "event-mark" the AT (vertical line) at the appropriate spot.

59

b. The systolic blood pressure reached a plateau (124-126/84 mmHg) at a ramp slope of 75-100 watts and remained flat for the remainder of the exercise.

c. The O_2/pulse flattened at 11 ml O_2/heart beat during the last 4 minutes of exercise (Figure 13). Although this value is the same as the patient's predicted normal, the "plateau effect" is distinctly abnormal, suggesting (along with the flat BP) that there is cardiac impairment. The O_2/pulse at the patient's WRmax is calculated as follows: $\dot{V}O_2$/HR = 1850 ml O_2/169 beats (per min) = 11.0 ml O_2/heart beat.

d. The heart rate reserve was normal:

HRR = 1 − [(169-67)/(201-67)] = 24%.

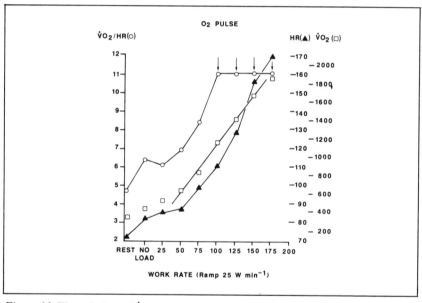

Figure 13. The relation of $\dot{V}O_2$, heart rate (HR), and O_2/pulse is shown to the work rate in graphic form. Arrows indicate a "plateau" of the O_2/pulse starting at a work rate of 100 watts and continuing until the end of exercise at 200 watts. This abnormal response suggests a reduced stroke volume. In addition, the event was accompanied by flattening of the systolic blood pressure at 124-126/84 mmHg.

Item 9.

Ventilation/Perfusion $(\dot{V}/\dot{Q})$ was normal:

a. The V_D/V_T dropped normally from 0.32 at rest to 0.16 at WRmax. The calculation at WRmax is made as follows:

$$V_D/V_T = \frac{PaCO_2 - P_ECO_2}{PaCO_2} = \frac{43 - 35.96}{43} = 0.16,$$

Where $P_ECO_2 = [\dot{V}CO_2/\dot{V}_E - (V_D\text{valve} \times f_b)] \times 0.863$
$= [2140 \text{ ml}/54.2 - (0.095 \times 30)] \times 0.863$
$= 35.96$

b. $P(A-a)O_2$ was normal at rest (7 torr) and also at WRmax (10 torr). The mild rise in the A-a O_2 difference is a normal response to exercise.

c. $P(a-ET)CO_2$ responded normally. The partial pressure difference between arterial and end-tidal CO_2 fell slightly from $+ 1.5$ torr at rest to zero at WRmax.

Item 10.

The patient gave a "thumbs down" signal at the end of the 11th minute on the mouthpiece (7th minute of ramp exercise). The physician had already instructed the exercise technician to terminate the test. When questioned later, the patient stated that she felt short of breath and lightheaded, as if she might faint.

Item 11.

The post-exercise EKG revealed a normal sinus rhythm and no ST-T wave abnormalities. The P waves became normal almost immediately during recovery. Blood pressure reverted to 104/82 mmHg within 2½ minutes. The lungs were clear (no wheezing) on auscultation. Examination of the heart revealed a *mid-systolic click,* immediately followed by a soft systolic murmur. Note that the cardiac findings were normal prior to the exercise test.

Item 12.

The reader is referred again to Table 1 to review the raw data on the computer printout. Also, go over the information in Chapter 7 one more time.

Item 13.

The completed exercise report form is shown in the next Chapter as the third case report (Exhibit 3).

Item 14.

The patient was referred to cardiology. **An echocardiogram confirmed the clinical impression of a mitral valve prolapse.** The exact nature of the impairment was explained to the patient. She was advised to avoid strenuous exercise and given a one year appointment for a follow-up examination.

CHAPTER 9
SELECTED CASE REPORTS

Six case reports are presented in detail, each one having been selected for different reasons. For all of these patients, however, **the one symptom in common was dyspnea.** Again, these reports emphasize the tremendous value of exercise testing in the differential diagnosis of dyspnea . . . **cardiac vs. pulmonary.**

Summary

Case 1.

Dyspnea in a young woman secondary to repeated lung resections for metastatic synovial sarcoma. The thoracic surgeon was informed when additional wedge resections were no longer advisable because of the development of a significant breathing limitation (See Exhibit 1).

Case 2.

Dyspnea on exertion in a young adult male following a severe chest injury and multiple pulmonary emboli. A disability evaluation was carried out, and the patient determined to be 100% disabled for his job as a policeman (See Exhibit 2).

Case 3.

Dyspnea and dizziness on heavy exertion in a young woman (college student) who had an unsuspected prolapsed mitral valve. Exercise testing indicated cardiac impairment. A cardiology referral was made. The diagnosis was confirmed by an echocardiogram (See Exhibit 3).

Case 4.

Dyspnea in a woman with severe anxiety. The patient was referred to a psychiatrist (See Exhibit 4).

Case 5.

Dyspnea (only on exertion) in an avid jogger with a known, hemodynamically stable aortic stenosis. A diagnosis was made of exercise induced asthma. Abnormal ST-segment changes occurred in the absence of angina. Definite limitations in exercise were recommended (See Exhibit 5).

Case 6.
Dyspnea and a rapid respiratory rate in a youth with a demand pacemaker (complete A-V heart block) and a fixed heart rate of 84/min. Insertion of a new pacemaker was advised (See Exhibit 6).

Case Reports

Case 1 (Exhibit 1)
This case report illustrates what happened physiologically to a young adult female when her lung volume was reduced by lobectomy and by repeated wedge resections for metastatic sarcoma over a period of 18 months. Exercise testing added a new, dynamic dimension by indicating when further lung surgery was no longer advisable.

History

The patient is a 24-year-old woman (nonsmoker) who was in excellent health prior to developing a synovial sarcoma of the knee with spread to the lungs. In October, 1983, she had surgical removal of the primary tumor and a left upper lobectomy, followed in 6 weeks by multiple wedge resections of fresh lung nodules. Spirometry and exercise testing were performed on three occasions starting on May 31, 1984, one day prior to resecting more small lung metastases. The tests were repeated on November 19, 1984, after which she again had wedge resections for additional malignant lung nodules. Following this operation, the patient had to reduce her daily exercise program because of dyspnea on exertion. The final testing was done on April 4, 1985. A thoracotomy was performed the next day to remove 6 new, sarcomatous lung nodules.

Laboratory Results (Exhibit 1)

The pulmonary function tests showed a progressive restrictive ventilatory defect with significant loss of FVC, FEV_1, and a consistently high FEV_1/FVC of 94-95%.

Comparing the first and last ramp tests at WRmax (Exhibit 1), the results of cycle exercise revealed the following abnormalities: (1) a loss of work capacity from 94% to 70%; (2) a striking decrease in the anaerobic threshold from 56% to 38%; (3) a fall in the breathing reserve from 43% to 23%; (4) a rise in the respiratory rate from 52/min to 65/min; (5) a fixation of V_T at 50% of the FVC; (6) an increase in the $P(A-a)O_2$ from 8 torr to 24 torr; (7) a rise in the V_D/V_T from 0.21 to 0.27; (8) a change in the $P(a-ET)CO_2$ from -2.0 torr to $+6.0$ torr; (9) a drop in the O_2/pulse from 10 ml to 8.0 ml/beat; and (1) a rise in the "R" from 1.16 at 160 watts to 1.23 at 140 watts. At WRmax there were negligible changes over the 10 month period in the pH, $PaCO_2$, HCO_3^-, V_T/FVC, heart rate reserve, blood pressure, and EKG.

63

PULMONARY FUNCTION AND EXERCISE DATA (CASE 1)*
Changes in Spirometric and Exercise Testing Data
as a Result of Repeated Lung Resections

	31 May, 1984	19 Nov., 1984	4 Apr., 1985	Trend
FVC	2.32 L (52%)	2.25 L (50%)	1.73 L (40%)	↓
FEV$_1$	2.22 L (61%)	2.13 L (59%)	1.63 L (47%)	↓
FEV$_1$/FVC	95%	95%	94%	⟷
MVV	107 L (84%)	100 L (78%)	79 L (63%)	↓
pH: Rest→WRmax	7.41→7.31	7.43→7.31	7.46→7.32	⟷
PO$_2$: Rest→WRmax	96→106	99→108	93→86	↓
PCO$_2$: Rest→WRmax	40→38	37→33	37→40	⟷
HCO$_3$: Rest→WRmax	24→18	24→16	27→20	⟷
"R": Rest→WRmax	0.88→1.16	0.92→1.19	0.91→1.23	⟷/↑
WC • WRmax	95%	88%	70%	↓
V̇O$_2$max (ml/kg/min)	31	29	23	↓
AT	56%	50%	38%	↓
BR • WRmax	43%	31%	23%	↓
f$_b$: Rest→WRmax	18→52	20→63	20→65	↑
V$_T$/FVC: Rest→WRmax	0.19→0.50	0.22→0.50	0.34→0.50	⟷
P(A-a)O$_2$: Rest→WRmax	8→8	12→12	13→24	↑
V$_D$/V$_T$: Rest→WRmax	0.38→0.21	0.34→0.11	0.36→0.27	↑
P(a-ET)CO$_2$: Rest→WRmax	+4→-2	+4→-1	+6→+6	↑
HRR • WRmax	30%	28%	31%	⟷
HR-AT	128	125	115	⟷
O$_2$/pulse: Rest→WRmax	10	9	8	↓
BP: Rest→WRmax	106/76→160/72	110/80→145/85	110/70→150/75	⟷
EKG:Rest→WRmax	Normal	Normal	Normal	⟷

*Female, age 24 years, height 175 cm, weight 55.7 kg; Dx: metastatic sarcoma to lungs.
Predicted V̇O$_2$max = 1840 ml, HRmax = 196 beats/min, O$_2$/pulse = 9.4 ml O$_2$/beat.

Exhibit 1

Summary and Conclusions

The results of serial pulmonary function studies (PFT's) and exercise tests over a 10-month period resemble those seen in advancing restrictive lung disease. Although the PFT's showed only moderate impairment, the V̇O$_2$AT fell below 40%! Thus unexpected finding suggests circulatory impairment which most likely is due to the loss of pulmonary vascular bed. The V̇O$_2$max decreased from 29 to 23 ml/kg/min, which according to Smith et al (Am Rev Respir Dis 129:730, 1984) puts the patient **above** 15 ml/kg/min, a level **below** which post-thoracotomy complications are much more likely to occur. The surgeon was informed of the findings. The patient is scheduled to return for re-testing as soon as she has recovered from her latest thoracotomy.

Case 2 (Exhibit 2)

The value of exercise testing in the **disability evaluation** of a young adult male is shown in this case report.

History

The patient is a 30-year-old policeman (nonsmoker) who sustained a crushing chest wall injury in an auto-truck accident in 1981. The following diagnoses were made: (1) bilateral, multiple rib fractures resulting in a flail chest; (2) hematoma of the lung; (3) deep venous thrombosis of the right leg; (4) multiple pulmonary emboli; (5) respiratory failure. He required a tracheotomy, was on mechanical ventilation for 25 days, and had a stormy course before recovery. He was discharged from the hospital on anticoagulant therapy after a total of 6 weeks. Six months following the accident he returned to his job but found that it was a struggle for him to perform any duties requiring physical activity. He was placed on bronchodilator therapy by his physician for "asthma" and continued working. Finally, in 1985 he collapsed while chasing a criminal.

The subject was referred to our exercise laboratory for evaluation of his disability. On physical examination he appeared to be healthy. The lungs were clear to percussion and auscultation. A healed tracheotomy scar was present. The heart tones were normal. He was wearing elastic stockings.

Laboratory Results

Pre-exercise pulmonary function tests (spirometry, flow volume loop, body plethysmography) showed a restrictive ventilatory defect. FVC=4.30 L (69%); FEV_1=3.24 L (68%); FEV_1/FVC=75%; TLC=6.50 L (76%); RV=1.92 L (84%); FRC=2.6 L (55%); MVV=82 L (49%). Following bronchodilator therapy by aerosol (alupent), improvement occurred in the flow rates. The FEV_1 increased +14%, the FEF_{25-75} +53%, and the PF +31%. The FVC was essentially unchanged at +3%. **The results of stress testing on the cycle ergometer are shown in Exhibit 2.** Be sure and review this data before proceeding.

Interpretation of Exercise Data

The patient was cooperative and made a good effort. He had no chest pain, dizziness or claudication. The exercise test was submaximal as determined by only a 2 mEq drop in HCO_3^- and a slight fall in the pH from 7.43 to 7.40. The patient stopped exercising because of severe shortness of breath.

The work capacity was reduced to 60%, and the anaerobic threshold (AT) was abnormally low at 36%. The heart rate at the AT was 112 beats/min. A marked breathing limitation was clearly evident by a breathing reserve of zero. The breathing pattern was characteristic of restrictive lung disease. The tidal volume became fixed early in exercise, thus the increasing $\dot{V}_E$ demanded by exercise was accomplished by a sharp

EXHIBIT 2

UNIVERSITY OF IOWA HOSPITALS & CLINICS   NAME: CASE 2

CARDIOPULMONARY EXERCISE LABORATORY   AGE: 30   SEX:M   HT:190 cm   WT: 110 kg

HOSPITAL NO: -----

DATE: 29 Apr. '85   REF.MD:

Chief complaint: severe exertional dyspnea and fatigue.

HISTORY: 30-yr-old policeman who sustained a severe chest wall injury Sept.13,1981, in an auto-truck accident. Dx's: bilateral rib fractures (flail chest); hematoma of lung; deep venous thrombosis of rt.leg; multiple pulmonary emboli; respiratory failure requiring mechanical ventilation. Returned to job 6 mos. later. Given bronchodilators for "asthma".

PFT's: FVC=4.3 L(69%); FEV_1=3.24 L(68%); FEV_1/FVC=75%;
TLC=6.5 L(76%); FRC=2.6 L(55%); RV=1.92 L(84%); MVV=82 L(49%).

Some response noted to bronchodilators: FEV_1 increased 14%.

EXERCISE TEST: Cycle ergometer with a ramp slope of 25 watts·min⁻¹

Predicted Values:

$\dot{V}O_2$max   3539 ml

HRmax   190 beats

O_2/HR 18.4 ml/beat

WRmax   257 watts

MVV   84 L

	pH	PO_2	PCO_2	HCO_3	"R"
Rest:	7.43	79	38	24	0.87
WRmax:	7.40	81	37	22	1.09

		NORMAL	PATIENT
WORK CAPACITY: $\dot{V}O_2$max/pred. $\dot{V}O_2$max	(2140/3539)=	>85%	60%
ANAEROBIC THRESHOLD: $\dot{V}O_2$AT/pred. $\dot{V}O_2$max	(1280/3539)=	>40%	36%
BREATHING RESERVE: $1-(\dot{V}_E$max/MVV); also MVV $-\dot{V}_E$max	1-(85/84)= (84-85)=	>30% ; >15 L	zero
f_b: Rest → WRmax		8 → 60/min	10 → 53 breaths
V_T/FVC: Rest → WRmax		0.15 → 0.60	0.27 → 0.37
$P(A-a)O_2$: Rest → WRmax			38 → 32
V_D/V_T: Rest → WRmax		0.35 → <0.25	0.34 → 0.32
$P(a-ET)CO_2$: Rest → WRmax		+ 2 → <0	+6.0 → +4.0
HR RESERVE: 1-[(HRmax-HRrest)/(HRpred.max-HRrest)]	1-[(145-87)/(190-87)]=		44%
HR-AT (heart beat @ AT)			112 beats/min
O_2/Pulse: Rest → WRmax			4.6 → 14.8 ml/beat
BLOOD PRESSURE:			120/90 → 210/100

EKG: Incomplete RBBB before, during and after exercise. 4mm "P" pulmonale waves appeared during exercise and cleared within 3 minutes after exercise.

REASON EXERCISE STOPPED: Shortness of breath. Patient stopped upon completion of 125-150 W.

INTERPRETATION: The patient was cooperative and made a good effort. He had no chest pain, dizziness or claudication. The exercise was submaximal (only 2 mEq drop in HCO_3). The work capacity and anaerobic threshold were low. There was a marked breathing limitation (breathing reserve was zero!). Abnormalities were present in the $P(A-a)O_2$, V_D/V_T, and $P(a-ET)CO_2$, indicating mismatching of ventilation and perfusion, i.e., dead space ventilation. The high HR reserve and reduced O_2/HR were consistent with the premature termination of the exercise. EKG: incomplete RBBB; "P" pulmonale waves appeared during exercise, then cleared in the recovery period. Mild diastolic hypertension was present. IMPRESSION: (1) Submaximal exercise test; (2) Low work capacity and low AT; (3) Marked breathing limitation, plus an increase in dead space ventilation (mismatching of $\dot{V}/\dot{Q}$); (4) Restrictive ventilatory defect with borderline response to bronchodilators; (5) The low AT, abnormal gas exchange and exercise induced pulmonary hypertension are most likely the result of the chest injury and pulmonary emboli in 1981. RECOMMEND: (1) Rule out recent pulmonary emboli; (2) Disability evaluation on the treadmill using a "target" heart rate of 112 beats/min.

SIGNATURE *Dmald c Juvala* MD

Copyright: 1985, D.C. ZAVALA, M.D.

Exhibit 2

rise in the respiratory rate. Abnormalities were present in the $P(A-a)O_2$, V_D/V_T, and $P(a-ET)CO_2$, indicating mismatching of ventilation and perfusion ($\dot{V}/\dot{Q}$). The high HR reserve (44%) and the reduced O_2/HR were consistent with the premature termination of exercise by the subject. The EKG showed an incomplete right bundle branch block before, during, and after exercise. "P" pulmonale waves appeared early in exercise, reached a height of 4 mm at WRmax, then cleared within 3 minutes after exercise. The systolic BP rose normally; however, diastolic hypertension was present (90 mmHg at rest and 100 mmHg at WRmax). Post-exercise spirometry showed essentially no change as compared to pre-exercise values.

Impression

(1) Submaximal exercise test; (2) Low work capacity; (3) Low anaerobic threshold; (4) Mismatching of ventilation and perfusion ($\dot{V}/\dot{Q}$), resulting in increased dead space ventilation; (5) Prominent "P" pulmonale waves during stress testing, suggesting exercise-induced pulmonary hypertension; (6) Significant breathing limitation with zero breathing reserve; (7) Restrictive ventilatory defect on PFT's with a borderline response to aerosolized bronchodilator; (8) Unfitness; (9) Diastolic hypertension, mild.

Summary of Exercise Test

This 30-year-old policeman demonstrated significant circulatory impairment due to **pulmonary vascular disease,** most likely the result of his crushing chest injury and multiple pulmonary emboli in 1981. The impression of exercise induced pulmonary hypertension should be investigated further and recent pulmonary emboli should be ruled out. Bronchodilators should be continued. A methacholine challenge test may be helpful.

Disability Evaluation

After complete recovery from the cycle exercise, the patient was exercised on the treadmill at zero grade. The predicted treadmill speed to put him at his "target" heart rate of 112 beats/min (under steady-state conditions) was calculated as follows:

$$0.40 \times METmax = 0.40 \times \frac{(2140/110)}{3.5} = 2.2 \text{ mph}$$

Upon testing, the correct speed proved to be 2.0 mph. Higher speeds on the treadmill (e.g., 2.5 mph) produced significantly positive values in the calculation of his $\dot{V}O_2$ (6'-3'), which indicated that the subject was not in a steady state. Using this data, it was determined that the patient could perform the following **continuous activity:** drive a car, use hand tools for light work, operate a riding lawn mower, walk 2.0 mph on level ground, and do sedentary jobs such as desk work, filing, etc. Based on this report, the patient was declared 100% disabled as a policeman. Currently, he has returned to college and is preparing to become a minister. He has declined further testing at this time.

Case 3 (Exhibit 3): Reported in detail in Chapter 8.

UNIVERSITY OF IOWA HOSPITALS & CLINICS

CARDIOPULMONARY EXERCISE LABORATORY

NAME: CASE 3   EXHIBIT 3

AGE: 19   SEX:Fe   HT: 170 cm WT: 58.6 kg.

HOSPITAL NO: -----

DATE: 27 Jan.'85 REF.MD:

HISTORY: Chief complaint of shortness of breath, lightheadedness and dizziness which occurs only during considerable exertion at ballet practice and never during light exercise. Normal physical examination: no wheezing, normal heart tones. Negative chest x-ray and normal EKG.

PFT's:
Normal spirometry: FVC = 3.82 L (87%): FEV_1 = 3.5 L (99%); FEV_1/FVC = 92%; MVV = 101 L (80%); DLco = 94%.

Predicted Values:

$\dot{V}O_2$max __1982 ml__

HRmax __201 beats__

O_2/HR __9.9 ml/beat__

WRmax __145 watts__

EXERCISE TEST: Cycle ergometer with a ramp slope of 25 watts·min^{-1}

	pH	PO_2	PCO_2	HCO_3	"R"
Rest:	7.42	94	38	25	0.79
WRmax:	7.30	99	43	21	1.16

MVV   101 L

	NORMAL	PATIENT
WORK CAPACITY: $\dot{V}O_2$max/pred. $\dot{V}O_2$max (1850/1982) = . . .	>85%	93%
ANAEROBIC THRESHOLD: $\dot{V}O_2$AT/pred. $\dot{V}O_2$max (1150/1982) = . .	>40%	58%
BREATHING RESERVE: 1-(54.2/101); (101-54.2) = 1-($\dot{V}_E$max/MVV); also MVV - $V_E$max . .	>30% ; >15 L	46%; 46.8 L
f_b: Rest→WRmax	8 →60/min	18 →30 breaths
V_T/FVC: Rest→WRmax	0.15 → 0.60	0.14→0.47
$P(A-a)O_2$: Rest→WRmax		7→10 torr
V_D/V_T: Rest→WRmax	0.35 →<0.25	0.32→0.16
$P(a-ET)CO_2$: Rest→WRmax	+2 →<0	+1.5→0
HR RESERVE: 1-[(169-67)/(201-67)] = 1-[(HRmax-HRrest)/(HRpred. max-HRrest)] . .		24%
HR-AT (heart beat @ AT)		109 beats/min
O_2/Pulse: Rest→WRmax Flat O_2/HR last 4 min of exercise (after 100 watts).		4.7 →11 ml/beat
BLOOD PRESSURE: Systolic BP remained flat after 100 watts!		102/84 →124/84

EKG: Mildly prominent "P" pulmonale waves at work rates above 100 watts.

REASON EXERCISE STOPPED: Dizziness, lightheadedness, breathlessness. Patient felt like she was going to faint. Exercise stopped upon completion of 150-175 watts.

INTERPRETATION: The patient was cooperative and made a good effort. The exercise was maximal (HCO_3 dropped 4 mEq at WRmax). The following parameters were normal: work capacity, anaerobic threshold, breathing reserve, and gas exchange (ventilation-perfusion). During the last 4 minutes of exercise (work rates above 100 watts) the following abnormalities occurred: (1) The O_2/HR flattened, suggesting a reduced stroke volume; (2) The systolic BP hit a plateau, also suggesting cardiac dysfunction; (3) slightly prominent "P" pulmonale waves appeared on the EKG, suggesting mild pulmonary hypertension. IMPRESSION: (1) Abnormal cardiac response to exercise at work loads above 100 watts; (2) Normal work capacity, anaerobic threshold and ventilatory response to exercise. NOTE: Immediately after exercise, exam of the heart revealed a mid-systolic click and a soft systolic murmur. The lungs were clear. These findings are consistent with the diagnosis of a PROLAPSED MITRAL VALVE.

RECOMMEND: Cardiology referral; echocardiogram.

Copyright: 1985, D.C. ZAVALA, M.D.   SIGNATURE _Donald C Zavala MD_

Exhibit 3

68

Cases 4-6 (Exhibits 4-6)

The complete report forms on these three interesting cases are shown in Exhibits 4-6. The author suggests that the reader review the patient's history and laboratory data first, then form your own conclusions before reading the interpretation and recommendations.

UNIVERSITY OF IOWA HOSPITALS & CLINICS
CARDIOPULMONARY EXERCISE LABORATORY

NAME: CASE 4.
EXHIBIT 4
AGE: 41   SEX:Fe   HT:175 cm   WT:81 kg
HOSPITAL NO: ----
DATE: 26 Apr.'85 REF.MD:

HISTORY: Gave vague history of shortness of breath walking one block. Has a lot of suppressed anxiety. Uses a one-arm crutch for no apparent physical reason. Hysterectomy 1981. Is a non-smoker. No wheezing on chest exam.

PFT's: Not cooperative. Results unreliable. FVC = 1.48 L (36%); FEV_1 = 1.03 L (32%); FEV_1/FVC = 69%. DLco = 85%. MVV = 102 L (89%).... made good effort here.

EXERCISE TEST: Cycle ergometer with a ramp slope of 25 watts·min^{-1}

Predicted Values:
$\dot{V}O_2$max ___1957 ml
HRmax ___179 beats
O_2/HR 10.8 ml/beat
WRmax ___135 watts

	pH	PO_2	PCO_2	HCO_3	"R"
Rest:	7.46	82	40	27	0.92
WRmax:	7.35	96	33	18	1.25

	MVV	102 L

	NORMAL	PATIENT
WORK CAPACITY: $\dot{V}O_2$max/pred.$\dot{V}O_2$max 1580/1957 = ...	>85%	81%
ANAEROBIC THRESHOLD: $\dot{V}O_2$AT/pred. $\dot{V}O_2$max 838/1957 = ...	>40%	43%
BREATHING RESERVE: 1−($\dot{V}_E$max/MVV); also MVV − $\dot{V}_E$max 1−(61/102) = 102−61= . . .	>30% ; >15 L	40%; 41 L
f_b: Rest → WRmax	8 → 60/min	16 → 34 breaths
V_T/FVC: Rest → WRmax	0.15 → 0.60	FVC not reliable
P(A − a)O_2: Rest → WRmax		21 → 23 torr
V_D/V_T: Rest → WRmax	0.35 → <0.25	0.33 → 0.05
P(a − ET)CO_2: Rest → WRmax	+ 2 → <0	+5.0 → −3.0 torr
HR RESERVE: 1−[(167-87)/(179-87)] = 1−[(HRmax-HRrest)/(HRpred. max-HRrest)] . .		13%
HR-AT (heart beat @ AT)		119 beats/min
O_2/Pulse: Rest → WRmax (pred.at WRmax: 9.2 → 10.8) . . .		3.0 → 9.5 ml/beat
BLOOD PRESSURE:		120/80 → 170/90

EKG: Normal throughout.

REASON EXERCISE STOPPED: Exhaustion. Patient stopped upon completion of 125-150 watts.

INTERPRETATION: The patient was surprisingly cooperative and made a good effort although she tried to control her breathing early in the exercise. She had no chest pain, dizziness, or claudication. The test was maximal as evidenced by a fall in the bicarbonate from 27 to 18 mEq, a drop in pH from 7.46 to 7.35, and an "R" of 1.25 at WRmax. The work capacity was slightly reduced, and the anaerobic threshold was a low normal. Breathing reserve and heart rate reserve were both normal. The O_2/pulse was a low normal. The P(A-a)O_2, V_D/V_T, and P(a-ET)CO_2 all responded normally to maximal stress, indicating good matching of ventilation/perfusion. The BP response was normal; there were no abnormal EKG changes.

IMPRESSION: (1) Normal cardiopulmonary response to maximal exercise with good gas exchange; (2) Deconditioning as evidenced by decreased work capacity, anaerobic threshold and O_2/HR.

RECOMMEND: (1) reassurance; (2) exercise program; (3) psychiatric referral.

Copyright: 1985, D.C. ZAVALA, M.D.   SIGNATURE _Donald C. Zavala, MD_

Exhibit 4

EXHIBIT 5

UNIVERSITY OF IOWA HOSPITALS & CLINICS   NAME: CASE 5

CARDIOPULMONARY EXERCISE LABORATORY   AGE: 37   SEX:M   HT: 173 cm WT: 71.0 kg.

HOSPITAL NO: -----

DATE:13 Nov.'84   REF.MD:

HISTORY: The patient has known aortic stenosis. Cardiac catheterization 1 mo. ago revealed no evidence of heart failure and no significant changes since 1982. The patient reports that since last summer severe dyspnea is occurring after 5 minutes of jogging. Indication for exercise testing: cause of dyspnea on exertion.

Predicted Values:

PFT's: FVC = 5.15 L (105%); FEV_1 = 3.67 L (96%); FEV_1/FVC = 71%, DLco = 80%;
MVV = 176 L (128%)
(Note: subject is an active jogger.)

$\dot{V}O_2$max 2626 ml

HRmax   183 beats

O_2/HR 16.7 ml/beat

EXERCISE TEST: Cycle ergometer with a ramp slope of 25·watts min^{-1}

WRmax   195 watts

	pH	PO_2	PCO_2	HCO_3	"R"
Rest:	7.43	92	41	26	0.84
WRmax:	7.32	102	34	17	1.22

MVV   176 L

	NORMAL	PATIENT
WORK CAPACITY: $\dot{V}O_2$max/pred. $\dot{V}O_2$max (2942/2626) = . . .	>85%	112%
ANAEROBIC THRESHOLD: $\dot{V}O_2$AT/pred. $\dot{V}O_2$max (1300/2626) =. .	>40%	50%
BREATHING RESERVE: 1- ($\dot{V}_E$max/MVV); also MVV - $V_E$max ·· 1-(108/176) ; (176-108) =	>30% ; >15 L	39%; 68 L
f_b: Rest→WRmax	8 → 60/min	14 → 38 breaths
V_T/FVC: Rest→WRmax	0.15 → 0.60	0.15→0.55
P(A - a)O_2: Rest→WRmax		12 →18 torr
V_D/V_T: Rest→WRmax	0.35 →<0.25	0.34 →0.11
P(a - ET)CO_2: Rest→WRmax . . . . 1-[(157-73)/(183-73)] =	+ 2 → <0	+3.0 →-1.0
HR RESERVE: 1-[(HRmax-HRrest)/(HRpred. max-HRrest)] ··		24%
HR-AT (heart beat @ AT)		112 beats/min
O_2/Pulse: Rest→WRmax		4.0 →17 ml/beat
BLOOD PRESSURE:		115/80 200/88

EKG: 3mm ST-segment depression with slight downslope (only during heavy exercise). No associated angina. No T-wave changes. Sinus rhythm.

REASON EXERCISE STOPPED: Exhaustion. Abnormal ST-segment changes and high R noted. Subject completed 225-250 watts.

INTERPRETATION: The subject was cooperative and made an excellent effort. He denied chest pain, dizziness, or claudication. The exercise was maximal with clear evidence of lactic acidosis (9 mEq drop in HCO_3). Normal results include the work capacity, anaerobic threshold, breathing reserve, heart rate reserve, O_2/pulse, and gas exchange. Normal progression of the blood pressure. Abnormal EKG changes with downward-sloping ST-segment depression of 3 mm at work rates over 150 watts (HR above 125/min). Ten minutes post-exercise, the patient developed bronchospasm with wheezing that was documented by spirometry. The nadir was reached at 20 minutes with a fall in the FVC of -15%, FEV_1 -20%, FEF_{25-75} -22%, and PF -33%, as compared to pre-exercise values. IMPRESSION: (1) Exercise induced asthma; (2) Mild aortic stenosis with no evidence of hemodynamic limitation; (3) Coronary artery disease. RECOMMEND: (1) Cardiology referral; (2) Stop jogging; (3) Avoid exertion that will produce a pulse rate above 125/min; (4) Bronchodilator therapy was not prescribed since subject is asymptomatic during rest and normal activity.

Copyright: 1985, D.C. ZAVALA, M.D.

SIGNATURE *Donald C Zavala* m.d.

Exhibit 5

70

UNIVERSITY OF IOWA HOSPITALS & CLINICS   NAME: CASE 6   EXHIBIT 6

CARDIOPULMONARY EXERCISE LABORATORY   AGE: 14 SEX: M HT: 158 cm WT: 58.6 kg

HOSPITAL NO: -----

DATE: 11 Dec.'84 REF.MD:

HISTORY: Chief complaint: increasing exertional dyspnea for 8 months. Patient has Noonan's syndrome. At age 5 months: surgical correction for coarctation of the aorta and a patent ductus arteriosus. At age 11 yrs: surgery for subvalvular (hypertrophic) and valvular aortic stenosis, insertion of a Bjork-Shiley valve, repair of a ventricular septal defect and placement of a demand pacemaker.

PFT's: FVC = 2.89 L(84%); FEV_1 = 2.67 L(91%); FEV_1/FVC = 92%; MVV = 110 L (108%)

Imp: normal spirometry.

EXERCISE TEST: Cycle ergometer with a ramp slope of 20 watts·min^{-1}

	pH	PO_2	PCO_2	HCO_3	"R"
Rest:	7.42	95	41	26	0.97
WRmax:	7.31	95	39	19	1.22

Predicted Values:

$\dot{V}O_2$max	2669 ml
HRmax	206 beats
O_2/HR	13 ml/beat
WRmax	218 watts
MVV	110 L

		NORMAL	PATIENT
WORK CAPACITY: $\dot{V}O_2$max/pred. $\dot{V}O_2$max	. . . .	>85%	58%
ANAEROBIC THRESHOLD: $\dot{V}O_2$AT/pred. $\dot{V}O_2$max	. . . .	>40%	37%
BREATHING RESERVE: 1−($\dot{V}_E$max/MVV); also MVV − $\dot{V}_E$max	. .	>30% ; >15 L	42%; 46 L
f_b: Rest→WRmax (diaphragm is being stimulated by pace-maker.	. . . . .	8→60/min	25→62 breaths
V_T/FVC: Rest→WRmax	. . . .	0.15 → 0.60	0.19→0.36
P(A−a)O_2: Rest→WRmax	. . . .		9→18 torr
V_D/V_T: Rest→WRmax	. . . .	0.35 → <0.25	0.32→0.24
P(a−ET)CO_2: Rest→WRmax	. . . .	+ 2 → <0	+5.0→0
HR RESERVE: 1−[(HRmax−HRrest)/(HRpred. max−HRrest)]	. .		Indeterminate (pacemaker)
HR−AT (heart beat @ AT)	. . . .		Indeterminate (pacemaker)
O_2/Pulse: Rest→WRmax	. . . .		Indeterminate (pacemaker)
BLOOD PRESSURE:			120/70→150/70

EKG: Complete A-V heart block. Pacemaker-induced contractions at 84 beats/min.

REASON EXERCISE STOPPED: Exhaustion. Subject completed 120-140 watts.

INTERPRETATION: The subject was cooperative and made a maximal effort. He had no chest pain, dizziness or claudication. The exercise was maximal (HCO_3 fell 7 mEq at WRmax). Breathing reserve was normal, however, the respiratory rate was abnormally high. A contributing factor to the high f_b was from electrical stimulation of the diaphragm by the patient's low-lying cardiac pacemaker (verified by fluoroscopy). P(A-a)O_2, V_D/V_T, and P(a-ET)CO_2 all responded normally to stress. The O_2/HR and HR reserve were indeterminate since the HR is fixed at 84/min. EKG: complete A-V heart block; pacemaker complexes set at 84/min. IMPRESSION: (1) Low work capacity and anaerobic threshold; (2) Complete A-V heart block with a demand ventricular pacemaker set at 84 beats/min; (3) Suspect insufficient cardiac output (fixed heart rate) to meet the demands of strenuous exercise; (4) High frequency of breathing, contributed by electrical stimulation of the diaphragm from the low-positioned cardiac pacemaker. RECOMMEND: Cardiology referral; replacement of the old pacemaker.

Copyright: 1985, D.C. ZAVALA, M.D.   SIGNATURE *Donald C. Zavala, M.D.*

Exhibit 6

CHAPTER 10
COMMENTS OF CLINICAL IMPORTANCE

Physiologic Changes During Exercise

The physiologic interactions during exercise are clearly described by Wasserman in his state-of-the-art article "Exercise Physiology in Health and Disease".[3] During incremental or ramp exercise the $\dot{V}_E$, $\dot{V}CO_2$, and $\dot{V}O_2$ all increase linearly with the work rate up to the *anaerobic threshold* at which point the $\dot{V}O_2$ increase remains linear with the power but the $\dot{V}_E$ and the $\dot{V}CO_2$ become non-linear with the $\dot{V}_E$ increasing even faster than the $\dot{V}CO_2$. Thus, R increases, $P_{ET}O_2$ increases, and $P_{ET}CO_2$ decreases. V_D increases slightly during progressive exercise, but there is a large increase in V_T with the end result being a decrease in the V_D/V_T. The $P(A-a)O_2$, which is one of the best indicators of the efficiency of gas exchange, normally decreases during moderate exercise but increases during heavy exercise.

Pathophysiologic Changes in COPD

Exercise performance in patients with chronic obstructive pulmonary disease (COPD) may be limited by abnormal pulmonary mechanics, respiratory muscle dysfunction and impaired gas exchange. As a result, the following pathophysiologic changes may occur:[49]

(1) A limitation in the expiratory flow of air, secondary to a reduction in the maximal static recoil pressure (Pst) of the lung.[50,51]

(2) A loss of breathing reserve as measured by 1-($V_E$max/observed MVV). In severe emphysema this value approaches zero at WRmax or even becomes negative; however, the ventilatory impairment may be less in chronic bronchitis.[25,39,50]

(3) A reduction in V_T/FVC at WRmax, often down to 47% as compared to a normal ratio of 55-60%.[50]

(4) A change in the pattern of breathing due to incoordination of the respiratory muscles. This abnormal breathing pattern may lead to

nonlinearity of the $\dot{V}_E$ at low and moderate work rates.[49,52,53]

(5) An increase during exercise in FRC, RV, and V_D/V_T.[49,54]

(6) An increase in the work of breathing.[55,56] In COPD patients at low levels of exercise, the respiratory muscles can consume 35-40% of the total $\dot{V}O_2$ as compared to 10-15% in normal subjects.

(7) A reduction in WRmax and $\dot{V}O_2$max.[57,58]

(8) A lowering of the maximal O_2/pulse; however, *the slope of the rise during progressive exercise is normal if there is no heart disease.*[39]

(9) A desaturation in arterial oxygen during exercise. This finding is commonly associated with a Dco below 55% predicted, an FEV_1 less than 45% of predicted, and pulmonary hypertension.[59-61]

(10) An impairment in the removal of CO_2, resulting in an increase in both $PaCO_2$ and in the partial pressure difference between arterial and end-tidal CO_2.[3,39]

(11) A higher level of acidosis (lower pH) during anaerobic exercise due to a combined metabolic and respiratory acidosis.[39]

(12) Unfitness, poor nutrition, and greater energy demands.[49]

(13) Cor pulmonale (severe COPD).[62-64]

(14) An altered perception of breathlessness.[49]

NOTE: Patients with far advanced COPD, severe hypoxemia, and hypercarbia most likely DO NOT NEED AN EXERCISE TEST. On the other hand, exercise testing (e.g., cycle, treadmill, 6 minute[65] or 12 minute walk[66]) may be very useful in symptomatic patients with mild to moderate or moderately severe COPD to check for the degree of ventilatory limitation, possible arterial desaturation, and the role that O_2 therapy may play (for those who desaturate) in improving exercise performance and exertional breathlessness.

Pathophysiologic Changes In Interstitial Lung Disease

Interstitial lung disease includes a wide spectrum of lung disorders such as ideopathic pulmonary fibrosis (IPF), sarcoidosis, eosinophilic granuloma, collagen vascular disease, silicosis, asbestosis, and many more. The following pathophysiologic changes may occur in any of these fibrotic disease processes:[67]

(1) A restrictive ventilatory defect with *reduced* lung volumes, lung compliance, vital capacity and FEV_1 with a normal or increased FEV_1/FVC ratio.[68] An obstructive component sometimes is seen, but in our experience this finding most commonly has been associated with cigarette smoking.

(2) Reduce compliance.[69]

(3) Increased elastic work of breathing.[67]

(4) Excessive ventilation for the degree of exercise.

(5) Abnormal breathing pattern characterized by a low V_T and high f_b, although the V_T/VC ratio remains normal.[70-72] During progressive exercise, $\dot{V}_T$max is reached early and from thereon $\dot{V}_E$ is achieved by a rapid rise in the rate of breathing ($V_T \times f_b = \dot{V}_E$).

(6) Mismatching of ventilation and perfusion with high and low $\dot{V}/\dot{Q}$ areas resulting in increased dead space ventilation (high V_D/V_T)[73, 74] and shunting.[75-77]

(7) Reduced diffusion across a thickened alveolar capillary membrane (accounts for up to 20% of gas exchange abnormality).[78]

(8) *During rest* in severe fibrosis: a reduced PaO_2, O_2 saturation, and Dco. *During exercise* in moderate to severe fibrosis: a progressive fall in PaO_2 and arterial O_2 saturation along with an increase in the A-aO_2 difference. Occasionally in early, mild disease, the resting arterial blood gases may improve during exercise.[78]

(9) Exercise induced pulmonary hypertension in advanced disease. In pulmonary vasculitis (e.g., scleroderma, eosinophilic granuloma)[79,80] the pulmonary artery pressure may rise with exercise even though spirometry is only mildly abnormal.

There is some question, and rightfully so, as to *the role that exercise testing should play in managing patients with interstitial lung disease.* After all, why carry out exercise testing in these individuals since the severity of lung pathology correlates reasonably well with the vital capacity, Dco, and the resting arterial blood gas values? Recently, Kelley and Daniele carefully reviewed the pathophysiology of pulmonary interstitial disease and gave several excellent reasons to selectively perform stress testing in this group of patients:[67]

(1) To determine the extent of arterial O_2 desaturation during exercise in patients with a resting Dco below 60% of predicted.

(2) To evaluate occupational impairment, i.e., the ability of the patient to perform his or her job.

(3) To appraise the response to therapy, especially in *complex* cases.

(4) To detect $\dot{V}/\dot{Q}$ mismatching in suspected *early* interstitial disease at which time the spirometry, resting arterial blood gas, and chest radiograph may all be normal. The Dco may be reduced.

(5) To help differentiate cardiac from pulmonary dyspnea in patients with combined cardiopulmonary disease.

(6) To assess patients who have dyspnea which is out of proportion to the results of their pulmonary function tests and arterial blood gases. *Small pulmonary emboli* must be considered in the differential diagnosis.

Anaerobic Threshold and the HR-AT

The anaerobic threshold (AT) lies just above the level of our usual daily work rate. Occasional spurts of energy, such as running up a flight of stairs, has essentially no effect on the AT. In fact, *a training effect* will not occur unless physical activity is carried out above the AT on a regular basis. In sedentary people, the AT is profoundly influenced by endurance training with a significant increase in the $\dot{V}O_2AT$, expressed as absolute $\dot{V}O_2$ or as a percentage of the $\dot{V}O_2max$.[81]

The heart rate at the Anaerobic Threshold (HR-AT) is a valuable bit of information. In non-ventilatory limited patients, the HR-AT can be used as a "target" in writing exercise prescriptions to start patients out on conditioning and rehabilitation programs. Subsequently, when a training effect is achieved, there will be a new "set-point" for the HR-AT with an appreciable increase in the O_2/pulse, primarily due to the increment in the $\dot{V}O_2$.

Rehabilitation

Intelligent, well motivated patients with strong family support make good candidates for rehabilitation. Also the age of the patient, the degree of illness, and any co-existing diseases are important factors.[82,83] The medical contraindications for rehabilitation are the same contraindications as those listed for exercise testing on page 6. Hodgkin and colleagues[83] have emphasized the benefits of pulmonary rehabilitation which are: (1) a reduction in symptoms and days spent in the hospital, (2) a reversal of anxiety-depression, (3) an increased ability to carry out daily activities including exercise, and (4) an improved quality of life. The same benefits may be achieved by cardiac rehabilitation.

In any rehabilitation program a reasonable question to ask of the exercise test is: "Why is the patient limited and to what degree is the limitation?" Comparative ergometric testing of a person's performance makes it possible to assess the limitation, to prescribe exact dosages of exercise, and to assure the success of a rehabilitation program. The concept of a training threshold was proposed by Karvonin and colleagues in 1957.[84] These investigators recognized that *insufficient training* does not help and, in fact, may lead to a loss of work capacity. *Excessive training* also leads to loss of capacity and negates the beneficial effects of exercise. The American Heart Association has long emphasized the importance of a GRADED EXERCISE CONDITIONING PROGRAM based on the physical status of the patient.[85] *Thus, there is the need for an exercise prescription ... one tailored to fit the patient's condition.*

At the University of Iowa Hospitals & Clinics, our rehabilitation program is divided into two sections: one for the cardiac patient and one for the pulmonary patient. In **cardiac rehabilitation** we use the patient's heart rate as a guide to exercise training. Likewise, a training heart rate is used in older "healthy" people who lead inactive life-styles. In the **ventilatory limited group,** the heart rate is of little or no value in writing an exercise prescription. Instead, other methods for prescribing exercise are employed as described below.

Exercise Workout, Prescriptions, Training, Medications

The Workout: As individuals, we are responsible for our own physical fitness. Nevertheless, healthy people can be helped tremendously by trained exercise group leaders* who can get a sedentary, normal adult into shape. Strong motivation is gained by group participation and by an enthusiastic exercise leader who sets a good example for others to follow.[86]

To be effective, the exercise must be carried out once daily at least 4 days/week, for a period of 20-30 minutes each session.[87] Like Gaul, the workout is divided into three parts: (1) the warm-up (10 minutes); (2) the main workout (20-30 minutes); and (3) the cool-down (5 minutes).[86] For the **warm-up,** low intensity exercises are appropriate, including stretching, flexing, walking or cycling at a low work rate. A reasonable target heart rate for the warm-up is an increase of 20 beats/minute over the resting pulse. In a similar fashion, very mild exercises are performed for the **cool-down** such as slow walking or pedaling the cycle at "no load" so that at the end of 5 minutes the pulse is below 100/minute.[86] Encouraging patients to take their own heart rates (radial, carotid or precordial sites) will improve their confidence in monitoring their exercise. For the **main workout,** an *optimal training heart rate* (for most healthy adults) is in the range of 140-160 beats/min. A *safe,* reasonable intensity for older adults is 120-140 beats/min. In Getchell's experience the training heart rate is a 75% elevation of the difference between the sitting and the maximal heart rate.[86] Prior to starting an exercise program, thorough evaluations, exercise testing, and individualized exercise prescriptions are recommended *for older, inactive adults, for people who have a medical problem, or for anyone who is at high risk to develop heart disease.*

Exercise Prescriptions: Walking, arm exercises, jogging and cycling are excellent forms of exercise. For deconditioned, older adults and for low-risk heart patients who do not have pulmonary impairment, our rehabilitation program consists of writing a prescription for the individual to start exercising just below his or her HR-AT for 20-30 minutes daily, a minimum of 4 times per week on separate days. Starting patients at this fairly light level of exertion will avoid undue stress and will insure that

*The American College of Sports Medicine has a certification program.

they can complete their exercise without terminating prematurely because of exhaustion and discomfort. Also, at the beginning of an exercise program, short bursts of more vigorous exercise are usually well tolerated by the subject. Subsequently, depending upon the physical condition and the response of the patient, the target heart rate may be increased periodically (e.g., 1 week initially, then every 2-3 weeks) by increments of 5 beats/minute until reaching an *optimal level of training* as discussed in the two sections immediately below.

Optimal Training: Without question, a maximal exercise test provides valuable information whereby an exercise prescription (as so well-stated by Franklin and colleagues) can be "adapted to the patient, rather than the patient to the prescription."[87] As recommended above, the *initial* target heart rate (at the beginning of the training program) should be just below the HR-AT, with increases being made as the conditioning progresses. To determine the *optimal intensity* for aerobic-exercise training (utilizing target heart rates) the following methods are used:

(1) 0.6-0.8 (HRmax-HRrest) + HR rest ....Karvonen[84]
(2) 70%-85% HRmax ....Hellerstein et al[88]
American Heart Assn.[89]
(3) 57-78% $\dot{V}O_2$ max ....Franklin & Hellerstein[87]
(4) 0.3-0.5 ($\dot{V}O_2$ max-$\dot{V}O_2$AT) + $\dot{V}O_2$AT .....Casaburi & Wasserman[90]

Currently we are using Casaburi and Wasserman's method and have not encountered any problems in overestimating the training heart rate. Note that their estimated level of optimal training (formula No. 4) is based on the subject's *anaerobic threshold* as well as the $\dot{V}O_2$ max. The following example is a review of the calculations for this method: Given a 50 year-old, "healthy" but sedentary male whose height $= 180$ cm, weight $= 82$ kg, measured $\dot{V}O_2$max $= 2250$ ml O_2/min, and $\dot{V}O_2$AT $= 1200$ ml 0_2/min, then his *optimal intensity* of exercise is a target heart rate which corresponds to 67%-77% of his $\dot{V}O_2$max.

Intensity of Exercise:

A useful guide to the intensity of exercise is the *rating of perceived exertion* (RPE) by Borg.[91] On a scale of 6 to 20: 9 is very light, 11 is light, 13 is somewhat hard, 15 is hard, 17 is very hard and 20 is very, very hard. Thus, for early cardiac rehabilitation an RPE of 11-12 would be appropriate, and later in training an RPE of 13 to 15 would correspond to 70%-85% of the HRmax or 57%-78% of the $\dot{V}O_2$max.[87,88,92] *For most myocardial infarction patients, however, the threshold intensity for exercise training lies in the range of 40-60% of the $\dot{V}O_2$max.*[93]

77

MI and CABGS Patients: Specific, detailed guidelines for an inpatient-outpatient rehabilitation program involving the myocardial infarction (MI) patient and the coronary artery bypass graft surgery (CABGS) patient are given in an excellent article by Metier, Pollock & Graves (J Cardiopulmonary Rehab 6:85-103, 1986). The authors point out that the CABGS patient usually has a faster and more vigorous start in exercise than the MI patient, however, range of motion exercises (upper extremity and trunk) must be avoided in the CABGS patient until the sternum becomes stable. Also chest discomfort from the operation must be distinguished from angina since unstable angina would preclude exercise. Normally, CABGS patients begin ambulation the first postoperative day and MI patients around 5 to 8 days after their infarction. **Early inpatient exercise** is normally performed at the 2-MET level (walking 1.5-2.0 mph) for both types of patients with the HRmax never more than 20 beats/min above the standing HR (Pollock ML, et al: *in* Heart Disease and Rehabilitation, 2nd ed., New York, John Wiley, 1986, 447-516). Telemetric monitoring of the EKG during exercise may provide highly useful information regarding potentially serious rhythm disturbances (ventricular and supraventricular dysrhythmias) and myocardial ischemia. Angina-limited patients must settle for a training heart rate of 5 beats/min below their angina threshold. At 4 to 8 weeks after the MI or CABGS, a symptom-limited, progressive exercise test may be performed to provide a sound basis for an **exercise prescription**. For the low risk cardiac patient, Metier et al favor the optimal training heart rate to be based on percent of the HRmax reserve (60%-85% [HRmax-HRrest] + HRrest). Zavala prefers to use the HR at the patient's anaerobic threshold (HR-AT), starting the exercise just below the HR-AT and progressing slowly to a desirable level above the anaerobic threshold based on the $\dot{V}O_2$ using the modified formula, $0.1\text{-}0.2 \, (\dot{V}O_2\text{max-}\dot{V}O_2\text{AT}) + \dot{V}O_2\text{AT}$. For low-risk patients who are at least 6 weeks post MI or CABGS, Metier and colleagues have had good results using a carefully graded Nautilus program. Candidates for this program must have an ejection fraction greater than 50%, a maximal work capacity of 7-8 METS, and a normal blood pressure response to stress.

Medications: Of special note is the fact that patients with *fixed heart rates* (pacemakers) benefit from modified exercise very much like patients with responsive heart rates.[94] Contrary to earlier beliefs, patients receiving *beta adrenergic blockers* will have a beneficial training effect from an exercise program even though there is attenuation of heart rate.[95-97] Hossack et al demonstrated that the regression of percent $\dot{V}O_2$max on percent HRmax is not changed by *propanolol*.[98] Also *diltiazem*, a calcium-channel blocker, will not alter the relationship of 57%-75% $\dot{V}O_2$max being proportional to 70%-85% HRmax.[99]

Ventilatory Limited Patients: In breathless patients with significant obstructive lung disease (FEV_1 < 1.2-1.4 L or FEV_1/FVC < 50%), selecting an optimal target heart rate may not be useful in planning their exercise program. Instead, alternate programs are recommended, the most useful of which are the following self-paced tests: (1) **a 6- or 12-minute walk test,** [65,66] which consists of walking as far as possible in 6 or 12 minutes on a level surface (shopping malls are ideal for this type of exercise). Subsequently, encouragement is given to gradually increase the distance walked in the given time period. From a practical standpoint this simple type of test is extremely useful in evaluating and improving the patient's exercise capacity, however, physiologic measurements are not made during the exercise; (2) **a level treadmill walk test,** starting at 1.0 mph for 6 or 12 minutes with the subject adjusting the rate of speed (Crockcroft, A: Practical Cardiol 12(4): 133,1986). Distance, heart rate, electrocardiograhic tracing, and oxygen saturation by ear oximetry are recorded. After a training program of gradually increasing the rates (still under control of the patient), significant improvement has been observed in the distances walked. Also in selected cases, ventilation and gas exchange can be measured with the patient breathing through a mouthpiece; (3) **a stationary bicycle self-paced test,** starting at "free-wheeling" (no load) for 6 to 12 minutes and gradually increasing at low work rates (e.g., 10-15 watts, constant load) as tolerated by the patient. This is an excellent exercise to use at home during inclement weather (e.g., wintertime in Iowa). Again, physiological measurements can be taken in selected cases with the patient on a mouthpiece.

For patients who are not so severely limited in their ventilation, the traditional progressive or ramp exercise test can be carried out on the cycle ergometer or treadmill and then a work level identified that requires a $\dot{V}_E$ which corresponds to approximately 50% to 60% of the patient's maximal $\dot{V}_E$.[86] Ideally for optimal training, any of the above exercises should be carried out daily, but at least 2 or 3 nonconsecutive days could be missed per week. Also as stated previously, supplemental nasal oxygen may be administered if the patient undergoes arterial O_2 desaturation.

Disability

When dealing with disability evaluations, we obtain the HR-AT on the cycle and then match it on the treadmill under steady-state conditions by having the subject walk level at a given rate of speed. We found that the initial belt speed (mph) to achieve the desired "target" heart rate is approximately 40% of the patient's METS at WRmax, i.e., $0.40 \times$ METmax = mph on the treadmill at zero grade. This estimated belt speed will put patients near their HR-AT (unpublished data by D. C. Zavala), at which point small adjustments can be made in the speed to give the

79

desired HR. Normally, steady state conditions can be reached within 3 minutes if the work rate is not too high. Observe that the treadmill test should not be done until the subject has fully recovered from the maximal exercise. The treadmill speed obtained at the target heart rate is a result that is easily understood by non-medical people. In addition, the rate of walking can be conveniently expressed as METS which then can be equated to other forms of *continuous* physical activity (Tables 2, 3). This type of disability evaluation does not provide an estimate for discontinuous or brief, intermittent work.

Arm Exercises

Walking, jogging, and cycling are traditional forms of exercise, however, **upper extremity exercises** also are beneficial. These exercises employ "towel-and-dowel," rings on a pegboard, arm weights, dumbbells, an arm ergometer or a set of ropes, pulleys and weights. For a given work load, arm work requires more energy than leg work because the muscle mass to work load is smaller.[101] For severe COPD patients, **supported** arm exercises are recommended as being more beneficial than **unsupported** arm exercises.[102] If low level, nonstrenuous upper extremity exercises are desired, then one rule-of-thumb is that the patient's heart rate is not permitted to rise more than 20 beats per minute from the resting rate.[101]

APPROXIMATE METABOLIC COST OF ACTIVITIES*

ACTIVITY	SPEED (level)	O_2 UPTAKE
WALKING	2 mph (3.2 km)	2 - 3 METS
WALKING	3 mph (4.8 km)	3 - 4 METS
WALKING	3.5 mph (5.6 km)	4 - 5 METS
WALKING	4 mph (6.4 km)	5 - 6 METS
WALKING	5 mph (8.0 km)	6 - 7 METS
JOGGING	5 mph (8.0 km)	7 - 8 METS
RUNNING	5.5 mph (8.9 km)	8 - 9 METS

*Data from Fox SM, Naughton JP, Gorman PA: Physical Activity and Cardiovascular Health. III, The exercise prescription; frequency and type of activity. Mod Concepts Cardiovas Dis 41: 6, June 1972.

Table 2

METABOLIC COSTS OF OCCUPATIONAL ACTIVITIES

	ACTIVITY	METS	$\dot{V}O_2$ ml/kg·min
Sitting:	**Light or Moderate Work**		
a.	Sitting at desk, writing, calculating etc.	1.5	4.25
b.	Driving a car	1.5	4.25
c.	Using hand tools, doing light assembly work, radio repair, etc.	1.8	5.30
d.	Driving a truck	1.8	5.30
e.	Working heavy levers, dredge, etc.	2.0	7.0
f.	Riding mower, etc., as individual work	2.5	8.75
g.	Sitting, for example, for a crane operator's job	2.5	8.75
h.	Driving heavy truck or trailer rig (must include getting on and off frequently and doing some arm work)	3.0	10.5
Standing:	**Moderate Work**		
a.	Standing quietly, assembling light or medium machine parts where speed is not a factor, working at own pace or a moderate rate	2.5	8.75
b.	Just standing, e.g., bartending	2.5	8.75
c.	Using hand tools (Gas station operator, other jobs where these are used, other than assembly work all day)	2.7	9.45
d.	Scrubbing, waxing, polishing (floors, walls, cars, windows)	2.7	9.45
e.	Assembling or repairing heavy machine parts such as farm machinery, plumbing, airplane motors, etc.	3.0	10.5
.	Light welding	3.0	10.5
.	Stocking shelves, packing or unpacking small or medium objects	3.0	10.5
.	Sanding floors with a power sander	3.0	10.5
.	Janitorial work	3.0	10.5
.	Kneeling or squatting doing light work	3.0	10.5

Table 3

(continued)

METABOLIC COSTS OF OCCUPATIONAL ACTIVITIES

ACTIVITY	METS	$\dot{V}O_2$ ml/kg.min
k. Assembling light or medium machine parts on assembly line or working with tools on line when objects appear at an approximate rate of 500 times a day or more	3.5	12.25
l. Working on assembly line when parts require lifting at about every five minutes or so; lifting involves only a few seconds at a time (parts weight 45 lbs. or less)	3.5	12.25
m. Same as "1" (parts weight over 45 lbs)	4.0	14.0
n. Cranking up dollies, hitching trailers, operating large levers, jacks, etc.	3.5	12.25
o. Pulling on wires, twisting cables, jerking on ropes, cables, etc., such as rewiring houses	3.5	12.25
p. Masonry, painting, paperhanging	4.0	14.0
Walking: Moderate Work		
a. Walking 3.0 mph	3.0	10.5
3.5 mph	4.0	14.0
b. Carrying trays, dishes, etc.	4.2	14.70
c. Walking involved in gas station mechanic work (changing tires, wrecker work, etc.)	4.5	15.75
Standing and/or Walking: Heavy Arm Work		
a. Lifting and carrying objects		
1. 20-44 lbs. (9-20 kg.)	4.5	15.75
2. 45-64 lbs. (20-29 kg.)	6.0	21.0
3. 65-84 lbs. (30-38 kg.)	7.5	26.25
4. 85-100 lbs. (39-45 kg.)	8.5	29.75
b. Heavy tools		
1. Pneumatic tools (jackhammers, drills, spades, tampers)	6.0	21.0
2. Shovel, pick, tunnel bar	8.0	28.0
c. Moving, pushing heavy objects, 75 lbs or more		
1. Desks, file cabinets, heavy stock furniture, such as moving van work. Also, pusing against heavy spring tension, as in boiler room, etc.	8.0	28.0

Table 3 (continued)

(continued)

METABOLIC COSTS OF OCCUPATIONAL ACTIVITIES

ACTIVITY	METS	$\dot{V}O_2$ ml/kg·min
2. Pushing a cart or dolly with objects weighing		
(a) less than 75 lbs.	4.2	14.70
(b) 75 lbs. or more	4.5	15.75
d. Other Responses		
1. Laying railroad track	7.0	24.5
2. Cutting trees-chopping wood		
(a) Automatically	3.0	10.5
(b) Hand axe or saw	5.5	19.25
e. Carpentry		
1. Activities involved in interior repair or remodeling (laying of tile, painting, etc.)	4.0	14.0
2. Building and finishing interior of house or garage	4.5	15.75
3. Putting in sidewalk (digging, carrying concrete, etc.)	5.0	17.5
4. Exterior remodeling or construction of house or garage (hammering, sawing, planing, etc.)	6.0	21.0
f. General heavy industrial labor		
1. Handyman work, some moving, some heavy work, such as shoveling, carpentry, etc.	5.0	17.5

Ref. Physician's Handbook for Evaluation of Cardiovascular and Physical Fitness, Tennessee Heart Association, Physical Exercise Committee, 1972, pgs. 41-43.

Table 3 (continued)

(Continued)
AVERAGE METABOLIC COSTS OF LEISURE ACTIVITIES

ACTIVITY	METS	$\overline{VO_2}$ ml/kg·min
Car driving, flying, model ship building	1.5	4.25
Darts, motorcycling (pleasure)	2.0	7.0
Model plane flying, mowing lawn (riding mower), power boating, shooting (rifle or pistol), shuffleboard, woodworking	2.5	8.75
Car washing, croquet, mechanical work on car	2.7	9.45
Billiards, pool, bowling, canoeing (2.5 mph), fishing (from boat, bank or ice), horseshoe pitching, plane building, shopping, wood cutting (power equipment)	3.0	10.5
Boat racing, driving a horse (sulky), horseback riding, ice boating, sailing (handling the boat)	3.5	12.25
Archery, baling hay, caring for horses, cycling (5.5 mph), farm work (sporadic), golf, table tennis, tetherball	4.0	14.0
Military marching, mowing lawn (power mower - not riding)	4.5	15.75
Gardening (weeding, hoeing, digging, spading) lawn work (raking, digging, filling), social dancing, softball or baseball (non-team, non-game, officiating)	5.0	17.5
Cycling (9.4 mph), fishing (wading in stream), hiking (cross-country), hunting, mowing lawn (push mower), shoveling (10/min. - 9 lbs.) softball (team game), square dancing, water skiing, water volleyball	6.0	21.0
Badminton, canoeing (4.0 mph) scuba diving, tennis	7.0	24.5
Basketball (non-game), basket ball (officiating), football (touch), motorcycling (endurance runs), mountain climbing, snow skiing, soccer (non-team)	8.0	28.0
Swimming Backstroke 40 yd./min.	8.0	28.0
Breaststroke 40 yd./min.	9.0	31.5
Crawl 45 yd./min.	9.5	33.25

Table 3 (continued)

(Continued)

AVERAGE METABOLIC COSTS OF LEISURE ACTIVITIES

ACTIVITY	METS	$\dot{V}O_2$ ml/kg·min
Cycling (13 mph), shoveling (10/min-14 lbs.)	9.0	31.5
Fencing, football (competition), gymnastics, snow sledding, tobogganing	10.0	35.0
Basketball (game play), canoeing or rowing (competition), hockey (ice), judo, handball, paddleball, soccer, space ball, squash, trampolining, wrestling	12.0	42.0
Shoveling (10/min. - 23 lbs.)	15.0	26.25

Ref. Physician's Handbook for Evaluation of Cardiovascular and Physical Fitness. Tennessee Heart Association, Physical Exercise Committee, 1972, pgs. 44-45.

Table 3 (continued)

Respiratory Muscle Exercises

In addition to the above variety of exercises, successful rehabilitation programs for COPD patients include diaphragmatic breathing exercises, pursed lip breathing, inspiratory resistance training, and nutritional repletion.[103-108] For endurance and strength training of the respiratory muscles, small devices such as PFLEX (HealthScan Products, Inc., Cedar Grove, NJ 07009) are commercially available which have a variable-sized orifice for inspiration and a one-way valve for expiration. Inspiratory muscle training should be done once or twice daily at an aperture that does not exhaust the patient. A training effect is achieved by decreasing the diameter of the inspiratory opening, thus increasing the inspiratory resistance. **On the other hand, hypercapneic patients may need respiratory muscle rest!**

Fitness

Physical fitness of the subject can be evaluated by looking at the exercise results of three measurements at WRmax: (1) work capacity, (2) anaerobic threshold, and (3) oxygen-pulse. High levels of these parameters equate with an excellent state of **fitness,** whereas low levels are found in states of deconditioning or unfitness. Often fitness is defined in terms of $\dot{V}O_2$max

85

and is expressed as O_2/kg/min.[1] Based on this measurement, the American Heart Association's fitness classification is shown in Table 4 (page 86). As for the O_2/pulse, a well-trained subject has a lower HR for a given VO_2 and consequently a higher O_2/pulse.

Unfitness goes hand-in-hand with cardiac or pulmonary disease, and the muscle wasting resulting from the patient's inactivity may further add to his or her disability. With this thought in mind, careful, prudent exercise may prove to be highly beneficial. For example, COPD patients report a decreased fear of exercise, increased tolerance of dyspnea, increased level of activity, and improved sleep. These benefits occur even though the results of spirometry remain unchanged.

Cardiorespiratory Fitness Classification*

WOMEN					
Age (yrs)	Maximal Oxygen Uptake (ml/kg/min)				
	Low	Fair	Average	Good	High
20-29	<24	24-30	31-37	38-48	49+
30-39	<20	20-27	28-33	34-44	45+
40-49	<17	17-23	24-30	31-41	42+
50-59	<15	15-20	21-27	28-37	38+
60-69	<13	13-17	18-23	24-34	35+

MEN					
Age (yrs)	Maximal Oxygen Uptake (ml/kg/min)				
	Low	Fair	Average	Good	High
20-29	<25	25-33	34-42	43-52	53+
30-39	<23	23-30	31-38	39-48	49+
40-49	<20	20-26	27-35	36-44	45+
50-59	<18	18-24	25-33	34-42	43+
60-69	<16	16-22	23-30	31-40	41+

*Exercise Testing and Training of Apparently Healthy Individuals: A Handbook for Physicians American Heart Association., 1972 p. 15

Table 4

Testing Cardiac Patients

A well recognized fact is that individuals with significant cardiac impairment characteristically develop high levels of blood lactate very early during graded exercise. The onset of lactic acidosis in these persons at low work rates is because of inadequate O_2 delivery to the muscle.[3] Nevertheless, in selected cardiac patients (Functional classes I-III), **exercise testing** using breath-by-breath analysis, offers the cardiologist a unique approach to gain information which may be extremely helpful in patient management. The patient's response to medical treatment or to cardiac surgery can be quantitated in terms of work capacity, anaerobic threshold, breathing reserve, gas exchange, heart rate reserve, oxygen-pulse, blood pressure, EKG, end-tidal O_2 and end-tidal CO_2.

Furthermore, carefully supervised exercise training (based on a "tailored" exercise prescription) is vital in the **rehabilitation** of the coronary heart disease patient, the post-myocardial infarction patient, and the patient who has had coronary angioplasty, coronary artery bypass graft surgery (CABGS) or valve replacement (Page 78). In reference to coronary artery disease, one should keep in mind that exercise testing does **not always** rule out this condition and that further definitive studies may be indicated on clinical grounds.

Cardiac Output

In routine clinical exercise testing, cardiac output is seldom measured, however, in a few selected cases, the physician may wish to obtain cardiac output during exercise testing. Both invasive and non-invasive methods have been developed which give reliable results, although the patient may be uncomfortable, especially when an arterial line is introduced or to a less extent when rebreathing CO_2.

The **direct, invasive approach** involves insertion of a Swan-Ganz catheter in the pulmonary artery. Hemodynamic monitoring includes the recording of pulmonary capillary wedge and right atrial pressures, the sampling of mixed venous blood for O_2 content and for the concentration of lactate, plus sampling of the radial artery for PO_2, PCO_2, pH, and O_2 content.[109,110] The **indirect or non-invasive technique** involves measurement of mixed expired CO_2 (F_ECO_2), minute ventilation ($\dot{V}_E$), carbon dioxide content in the arterial blood ($CaCO_2$), and the carbon dioxide content of the mixed venous blood. Many studies in normal individuals have shown that estimation of cardiac output without blood sampling is accurate.[111,112] **The steady-state cardiac output,** which uses the Fick principle and involves rebreathing CO_2 until equilibrium is reached, is described in detail by Jones.[1] A brief summary of the calculations involved is shown below:

$$C.O. = \cfrac{\overset{\displaystyle \overbrace{}^{\textstyle F_ECO_2 \times \dot{V}_E \text{ (STPD)} \times 10^3}}{\dot{V}CO_2}}{\underset{\underbrace{\phantom{C(\bar{v} - a) CO_2}}}{C(\bar{v} - a)\,CO_2}}$$

Arterial blood gas sample
Rebreathing bag sample (5-liter bag with 9-15% CO_2 in O_2)

Example of calculation: If the $\dot{V}CO_2$ is 2841 ml/min, the $PaCO_2$ is 27 torr and the $P\bar{v}CO_2$ is 72 torr (patient exercising at maximum effort) then,

log $CaCO_2$ = 0.396 × log (nl) $PaCO_2$ + 2.4 (antilog = 40.6 ml/100 ml × 10);

log $C\bar{v}CO_2$ = 0.396 × log (nl) $P\bar{v}CO_2$ + 2.4 (antilog = 59.9 ml/100 ml × 10);

Then,

$$C.O. = \frac{2841}{599 - 406} = \frac{2841}{193} = 14.7 \text{ liters/min;}$$

$$\text{Stroke volume} = \frac{14,700}{170} = 86 \text{ ml.}$$

HR

Heart Failure

As discussed previously, the patient's *cardiac status* can be assessed by observing the electrocardiogram, blood pressure, O_2/pulse and heart rate reserve during maximal exercise. On the other hand, the severity of *chronic cardiac failure* can be evaluated from the determination of $\dot{V}O_2$max and $\dot{V}O_2$AT. Based on the patient's $\dot{V}O_2$max (ml O_2/min/kg), Weber and colleagues classified the degree of cardiac failure as follows:[95]

CLASS	DEGREE OF HEART FAILURE	$\dot{V}O_2$max
Class A	no failure to mild failure	>20 ml O_2/kg/min
Class B	mild to moderate failure	16-20 ml O_2/kg/min
Class C	moderate to severe failure	10-15 ml O_2/kg/min
Class D	severe failure	6-9 ml O_2/kg/min
Class E	lactate produced at rest	6 ml O_2/kg/min

Testing for Exercise Induced Asthma

Patients with exercise induced asthma should respond to an inhalation challenge with histamine or methacholine.[113] Occasionally, however, it is useful to test patients suspected of having this bothersome syndrome on the treadmill (the preferred method of exercise in this instance) since the whole body is involved in movement, and the $\dot{V}O_2max$ is at least 10% higher than on the cycle. The belt speed on the treadmill is started at 2 mph and increased quickly to the subject's fastest (yet tolerable) walking rate. At this point, the speed is kept constant (usually 3.0–4.0 mph), but the grade is increased 3 degrees every minute until the patient reaches a heart rate of 80-90% of the predicted HRmax (220 − age [yrs]). This work rate is held for 6 minutes. Often the patients being tested are teenagers or young adults who, as a group, bear a near-maximal heart rate without difficulty. The only measurements taken are the pulse, blood pressure, O_2 saturation (by ear oximeter) and a 3-lead EKG with placements made at the angle of the right scapula, at the fifth interspace along the left anterior axillary line, and at the forehead. A 12-lead EKG is used if the subject is over 45 years old, has diabetes or a history of heart disease. Note that dry, compressed air may maximize the subject's degree of bronchospasm.[113]

The catecholamines released during exercise offer some protection against bronchospasm, therefore, spirometry is carried out at 5-10 minute intervals post exercise for a period of 20-30 minutes. The test is **positive for exercise induced asthma** if the FEV_1 decreases 20% or more and is **suggestive** if the FEV_1 drops 15-19%, as compared to pre-exercise levels. One also may look for evidence of lung hyperinflation with increases in RV, FRC, and TLC.[114-116] And finally, although exercise-induced anaphylaxis (urticaria, shock) is a rare event,[117-119] resuscitation equipment, epinephrine and inhaled beta-sympathomimetic agents should be on hand.[113]

Testing Obese Patients

Bariatric surgeons are beginning to request exercise testing on morbidly obese persons who weigh 200% or more than their ideal weight. The purpose of the exercise test is to determine which of these grossly overweight patients are safe candidates for gastric bypass, which are at higher risk, and which should have their surgery delayed until they are in better condition. Zavala and Printen reported on the requirements that they established for such an individual to be acceptable for operation.[28] **The patient must be able to walk level on a treadmill at 2 mph for 6 minutes without developing metabolic (lactic) acidosis with an "R" above 1.0.**

There are some unique problems in exercising morbidly obese patients. The ordinary seat on a cycle ergometer is too small, and a sling-type seat causes the subject to slide forward. On a treadmill, there is danger of injury since these huge people are awkward in their movements. Also good quality EKG tracings are difficult to obtain, especially on a treadmill. Another important factor is that patient motivation to carry out strenuous exercise is low.

Obese patients pay a terrible price for work! They require extraordinary amounts of O_2 to meet the metabolic requirements for a given work rate, thus, the heavier the person, the higher the $\dot{V}O_2$.[3] In our laboratory, we have observed super-obese patients (over 200 kg) who had oxygen uptakes of 3 liters or more, walking only 2 mph on the treadmill at zero elevation. Other characteristic physiologic phenomena for this group of unfortunate, overweight individuals are a low PaO_2 (with an increased A-a O_2 difference) and an elevated V_D/V_T at **rest**. These findings are due to $\dot{V}/\dot{Q}$ mismatching secondary to microatelectasis at the lung bases and are corrected by **exercise**.

Testing for O_2 Desaturation

Important information can be obtained simply by exercising the patient on a cycle or treadmill while monitoring the $SaO_2\%$ with an ear or pulse oximeter. The subject is not connected to a mouthpiece, and arterial blood gases are optional. A drop in the O_2 saturation of 5% (e.g., from 96% to 91%) or a fall below 90% is considered to be significant. The exercise should be terminated if the $SaO_2\%$ declines below 86%. At this level the O_2 saturation equates to a PaO_2 of 51-56 torr depending upon the pH (7.3 − 7.4). The finding of arterial desaturation indicates mismatching of ventilation:perfusion. Concomitant abnormalities may be observed in the V_D/V_T, $P(A-a)O_2$, and $P(a-ET)CO_2$, but obtaining these measurements requires that the subject be on a mouthpiece and that arterial blood gases are drawn.

Testing for Basal Oxygen Uptake

The **same exercise system** used for stress testing also can be utilized to carry out metabolic measurements under basal conditions! This intriguing approach involves the application of vastly improved equipment to revive an old test, formerly called the BMR or basal metabolic rate. The development of sophisticated methods to quantitate thyroid function (T_3, T_4, TSH) plus previous problems in measuring basal $\dot{V}O_2$, virtually put the concept of the "old" BMR into "mothballs". Based on the work of Lim and colleagues it now appears that basal oxygen uptake (ml O_2/kg/min) is indeed a sensitive index of the metabolic effects of thyroid hormones.[120] Recently these investigators found that BMR tests by modern methods of measurement (using the breath-by-breath analyzer) could be used with accuracy to follow the effect of therapy in patients with hyper- or hypothyroidism. They also observed that basal O_2 uptake was useful in guiding treatment for patients with thyroid hormone resistance and in assessing patients with the low T_3 syndrome associated with chronic renal failure or other non-thyroid illnesses.[121,122]

Ideally, patients should be tested during morning hours after an overnight fast. After resting comfortably in a semi-recumbent position for

90

½ hour, measurements are taken for 10 minutes and the mean values calculated.[28] For quality control of the "BMR", the expired air during the test is collected in a Douglas bag, meteorological balloon or Tissot for separate measurement of O_2 uptake and CO_2 production. Care must be taken to avoid a full bladder, tight noseclip, poorly fitting mouthpiece, awkward posture, unexpected sounds, ingested stimulants or depressants, muscular movement and anxiety.

Quality Control

The manufacturers and distributors of exercise systems have their own instructions to operate the equipment, however, much of the methodology is similar:

1) Information is fed into the computer regarding the patient (name, age, sex, weight, height, identification number, date, etc.) and the environment (room temperature, barometric pressure, relative humidity).
2) The O_2 and CO_2 analyzers are adjusted with known concentrations of dry gas.
3) The pneumotachometer (or its equivalent) is standardized with given volumes of room air, using a 3.0 liter super-syringe.
4) For breath-by-breath measurements, the response time of the O_2 and CO_2 analyzers must be determined, and the phase delay (between the flow signal and the gas signals) carefully checked and aligned.
5) The type of exercise test is entered into the computer:
   a. for the cycle ergometer, enter the work rate for a ramp or a 1-minute incremental exercise test. Don't forget to start each test with 2 minutes of rest and 2 minutes of unloaded pedalling.
   b. for the treadmill, enter the speed, grade and time span of each work rate. As an alternative, in some systems one simply may enter the name of the exercise protocol, e.g., Bruce protocol.

These routine, pre-procedural steps are essential. **In addition, daily records should be kept of the calibration of the exercise equipment.**

Quality control for your exercise system can be further assured by periodically exercising a trained subject (who has known values) under steady state conditions and also to WRmax. If such a person is not available, then you, another physician or one of the exercise technicians can be tested. The results obtained on the untrained person can be verified by the consistency of data obtained on repeated testing (done of different days) and by retesting this individual in another exercise laboratory.

At The University of Iowa, the following maneuvers for quality control are performed:

1) **a 50 watt constant-load exercise test on the cycle ergometer for 6**

91

minutes. Within 2-3 minutes, the test subject should enter a steady state which can be confirmed by a zero or near zero value for the $\triangle \dot{V}O_2$ (6'-3'). An average is taken of the computer's print-out data for the last 2 minutes of the exercise and compared with a bag sample of expired air collected during the same period of time and measured independently for $\dot{V}_E$, $\dot{V}O_2$, $\dot{V}CO_2$ and R (see equations, page   ). The steady state results of a healthy person are remarkably constant, providing the life style of that individual does not change. It is worthwhile to note that the **steady-state VO_2** of the test subject usually compares reasonably well with the predicted O_2 uptake calculated from Wasserman's quasi-steady-state equation[3]:

pred.$\dot{V}O_2$ (ml/min) = 5.8 × wt (kg) + 151 + [10.1 × watts].

2) **a 25 or 30 watt ramp or incremental exercise test on the cycle ergometer to WRmax.** Never do additional exercise testing on the same person immediately following a maximal test.

NOTE: Do not forget that your exercise programs come from "master" tapes at the various companies and that "glitches" occasionally occur. Consequently, always check out a new or revised tape as described above *before* using it on a patient.

SUMMARY

A well-equipped exercise laboratory with computerized techniques for breath-by-breath or mixing chamber measurements should have both a cycle ergometer and a treadmill. The preferred approach, following preliminary evaluation and preparation of the subject, is to initially stress the individual on a cycle using a ramp test or 1-minute incremental exercise to exhaustion. Occasionally, there are patients who cannot pedal a bicycle but perform reasonably well on a treadmill. In selected cases, constant-load exercise is helpful. Arterial blood gas samples before and during exercise will add highly useful information and are considered to be an integral part of the test.

A large amount of data will be generated in a short period of time whereby the patient's cardiovascular and respiratory systems can be appraised in meeting the gas-exchange requirements of exercise. Clinically, this information is useful for: (1) diagnostic purposes; (2) disability evaluations; (3) rehabilitation work-ups; (4) checking responses to therapy; and (5) assessing degrees of impairment and degrees of fitness.

In conclusion, exercise physiology is a fascinating, challenging field of study which has graduated from the arena of the physiologist into the sphere of the practicing physician. The importance of its role in clinical medicine and especially in the management of selected patients will, I am sure, increase rather rapidly. **Indeed, we owe a great deal to our friend, the exercise physiologist.**

REFERENCES

(1) Jones NL, Campbell EJM: *Clinical Exercise Testing.* 2nd Edition. Philadelphia, W.B. Saunders, 1980.

(2) Whipp BJ: Bioenergetics and gas exchange, Lecture delivered at the International Symposium on Exercise in Cardiac and Pulmonary Rehabilitation, Cambridge, MA, April 17, 1979.

(3) Wasserman K, Whipp BJ: Exercise physiology in health and disease. Am Rev Resp Dis 112:219-249, 1975.

(4) Wasserman K, Whipp BJ, Koval SN, Beaver WL: Anaerobic threshold and respiratory gas exchange during exercise. J Appl Physiol 35:236-243, 1973.

(5) Davis JA, Vodak P, Wilmore JH, Vodak J, Kurtz P: Anaerobic threshold and maximal oxygen uptake for three modes of exercise. J Appl Physiol 41:544-550, 1976.

(6) Karlsson J, Diamant B, Saltin B: Muscle metabolites during submaximal and maximal exercise in man. Scand J Clin Lab Invest 26:385-394, 1970.

(7) Wasserman K: The anaerobic threshold measurement to evaluate exercise performance. Am Rev Respir Dis 129:Suppl S35-S40, 1984.

(8) Wasserman K: Dyspnea on exertion. JAMA 248(16):2039-2043, 1982.

(9) Rochmis P, Blackburn H: Exercise tests: A survey of procedures, safety, and litigation experience in approximately 170,000 tests. JAMA 217(8):1061-1066, 1971.

(10) Hansen JE: Exercise testing. *In* Pulmonary Function Testing, Guidelines and Controversies. Academic Press, Inc., 1982, 259-279.

(11) Beaver WL, Wasserman K, Whipp BJ: On-line computer analysis and breath-by-breath graphical display of exercise function tests. J Appl Physiol 34:128-132, 1973.

(12) Sue DY, Hansen JE, Blais M, Wasserman K: Measurement and analysis of gas exchange during exercise using a programmable calculator. J Appl Physiol: Respirat Environ Exercise Physiol 49(3):456-461, 1980.

(13) Smodlaka VN: Treadmill vs bicycle ergometer. *In* Ergometry: Basics of Exercise Testing, Mellerowicz HM and Smodlaka VN (Eds.), Baltimore and Munich, Urban and Schwarzenberg, 1981.

(14) Stuart RJ, Ellestad MH: National survey of exercise stress testing facilities. Chest 77:94-97, 1980.

(15) Saunders NA, Powles ACP, Rebuck AS: Ear oximetry: Accuracy and practicability in the assessment of arterial oxygenation. Am Rev Respir Dis 113:745-749, 1976.

(16) Seldinger SI: Catheter replacement of the needle in percutaneous arteriography: A new technique. Acta Radiol (Stockh) 39:368, 376, 1953.

(17) Patterson JA, Naughton J, Pietras RJ, Gunnar RM: Treadmill exercise in assessment of the functional capacity of patients with cardiac disease. Am J Cardiol 30:757-762, 1972.

(18) Balke B, Ware RW: An experimental study of "physical fitness" of Air Force personnel. U.S. Armed Forces Med J 10:675-688, 1959.

(19) Bruce RA, Blackman JR, Jones JW: Exercise testing in adult normal subjects and cardiac patients. Pediatrics 32:742-755, 1963.

(20) Froelicher VF, Brammell H, Davis G, Noguera I, Stewart A, Lancaster MC: A comparison of the reproducibility and physiologic response to three maximal treadmill protocols. Chest 65(5):512-517, 1974.

(21) Cumming GR, Alexander WD: The calibration of bicycle ergometers. Can J Physiol Pharmacol 46:917-919, 1968.

(22) Davis JA, Whipp BJ, Lamarra N, Huntsman DJ, Frank MH, Wasserman K: Effect of ramp slope on determination of aerobic parameters from the ramp exercise test. Med and Sci in Sports and Exerc 14(5):339-343, 1982.

(23) Whipp BJ, Davis JA, Torres F, Wasserman K: A test to determine parameters of aerobic function during exercise. J Appl Physiol: Respirat Environ Exercise Physiol 50:217-221, 1981.

(24) Bell CW, Kass I, Hodgkin JE: Exercise conditioning. *In* Pulmonary Rehabilitation: Guidelines to Success. (Eds.) Hodgkin JE, Zorn EG, Connor GL; Boston, London, Sydney, Toronto, Butterworth Publishers, 1984, p. 201.

(25) Hansen JE, Sue DY, Wasserman K: Predicted values for clinical exercise testing. Am Rev Respir Dis 129:Suppl S49-S55, 1984.

(26) Bruce RA, Kusumi F, Hosmer D: Maximal oxygen uptake and normographic assessment of functional aerobic impairment in cardiovascular disease. Am Heart J 85:546-562, 1973.

(27) Wasserman K, Hansen JE, Sue DY, Whipp BJ: Principles of Exericse Testing and Interpretation. Philadephia, Lea and Febiger, 1986.

(28) Zavala DC, Printen KJ: Basal and exercise tests on morbidly obese patients before and after gastric bypass. Surgery 95 (2):221-229, 1984.

(29) Shephard RJ: Endurance fitness. Toronto, University of Toronto Press, 1969.

(30) Astrand P: Human physical fitness, with special reference to sex and age. Physiol Rev 36(Suppl. 2):307-335, 1956.

(31) Astrand I: Aerobic work capacity in men and women with special reference to age. Acta Physiol Scand 49 (Suppl 196): 1-92, 1960.

(32) Lange-Anderson K, Shephard RJ, Denolin H, Varnauskas E, Masironi R: Fundamentals of exercise testing. World Health Organization, Geneva, 1971.

(33) Spiro SG, Holm HL, Edwards RHT, Pride NB: An analysis of the physiological strain of submaximal exercise in patients with chronic obstructive bronchitis. Thorax 30: 415-425, 1975.

(34) Freedman S: Sustained maximal voluntary ventilation. Resp Physiol 8: 230-244, 1970.

(35) Clark TJH, Freedman S, Campbell EJM: The ventilatory capacity of patients with chronic airway obstruction. Clin Sci 36: 307-316, 1969.

(36) Sutton JR, Jones NL: Exercise testing in health and disease. Monograph for Phase III, Cardiorespiratory Unit, McMaster University, Hamilton, Ontario, Canada, Jan. 1978.

(37) Wasserman K, Whipp BJ, Davis JA: Respiratory physiology of exercise: Metabolsim, gas exchange, and ventilatory control. In International Review of Physiology, Respiratory Physiology III, vol. 23, Edited by John G. Widdecombe, Baltimore, University Park Press, 1981.

(38) Wasserman K, McIlroy MB: Detecting the threshold of anaerobic metabolism in cardiac patients during exercise. Am J Cardiol 14:844-852, 1964.

(39) Nery LE, Wasserman K, French W, Oren A, Davis JA: Contrasting cardiovascular and respiratory responses to exercise in mitral valve and chronic obstructive pulmonary diseases. Chest 83:446-453, 1983.

(40) Furuike AN, Sue DY, Hansen JE, Wasserman K: Comparison of physiological dead space/tidal volume ratio and alveolar-arterial PO_2 difference during incremental and constant work exercise. Am Rev Respir Dis 126:579-583, 1982.

(41) Cotes JE: Lung Function, 4th edition, 1979, Oxford, London, Edinburgh, Melbourne, Blackwell Scientific Publications, pp. 16-18.

(42) Wilmore JH, Costill DL: Adequacy of Haldane transformation in the computation of exercise VO_2 in man. J Appl Physiol 35:85-89, 1973.

(43) Bruce RA: Normal values for VO_2 and the VO_2-HR relationship. Am Rev Respir Dis 129:Suppl S41-S43, 1984.

(44) Jones NL, McHardy GJR, Naimark A, Campbell EJM: Physiological dead space and alveolar-arterial gas pressure differences during exercise. Clin Sci 31:19-29, 1966.

(45) Jones NL: Normal values for pulmonary gas exchange during exercise. Am Rev Respir Dis 129:Suppl S44-S46, 1984.

(46) Whipp BJ, Wasserman K: Alveolar-arterial gas tension differences during graded exercise. J Appl Physiol 27:361-365, 1969.

(47) Shepard RH, Campbell EJM, Martin HB, Enns T: Factors affecting pulmonary dead space as measured by single breath analysis. Am J Physiol 183:661, 1955.

(48) Bradley CA, Harris EA, Seelye ER, Whitlock RML: Gas exchange during exercise in healthy poeple. I. The physiological dead space volume. Clin Sci Mol Med 51:323-333, 1976.

(49) Loke J, Mahler DA, Paul Man SF, Wiedemann HP, Matthay RA: Exercise impairment in chronic obstructive pulmonary disease. Clinics in Chest Medicine 5 (No. 1): 121-143, 1984.

(50) Potter WA, Olafsson S, Hyatt RE: Ventilatory mechanics and expiratory flow limitation during exercise in patients with obstructive lung disease. J Clin Invest 50: 910-919, 1971.

(51) Gibson GJ, Pride NB: Lung distensibility: The static pressure-volume curve of the lungs and its use in clinical assessment. Br J Dis Chest 70: 143-184, 1976.

(52) Ashutosh K, Gilbert R, Auchincloss JH Jr, Peppi D: Asynchronous breathing movements in patients with chronic obstructive pulmonary disease. Chest 67: 553-557, 1975.

(53) Sharp JT, Goldberg NB, Druz WS, Fishman HC, Danon J: Thoracoabdominal motion in chronic obstructive pulmonary disease. Am Rev Respir Dis 115: 47-56, 1977.

(54) Stubbing DG, Pengelly LD, Morse JLC, Jones N: Pulmonary mechanics during exercise in normal males. J Appl Physiol: Respirat Environ Exercise Physiol 49: 506-510, 1980.

(55) Levison H, Cherniak RM: Ventilatory cost of exercise in chronic obstructive pulmonary disease. J Appl Physiol 25: 21-27, 1968.

(56) Field S, Kelly SM, Macklem PT: The oxygen cost of breathing in patients with cardiorespiratory disease. Am Rev Respir Dis 126: 9-13, 1982

(57) Pierce AK, Taylor HF, Archer RK, Miller WF: Responses to exercise training in patients with emphysema. Arch Intern Med 113: 28-36, 1964.

(58) Minh VD, Lee HM, Vasquez P, Shepard JW, Bell JW: Relation of $\dot{V}O_2$max to cardiopulmonary function in patients with chronic obstructive lung disease. Bull Eur Physiopathol Respir 15: 359-375, 1979.

(59) Minh VD, Lee HM, Dolan GF, Light RW, Bell J, Vasquez P: Hypoxemia during exercise in patients with chronic obstructive pulmonary disease. Am Rev Respir Dis 120: 787-794, 1979.

(60) Owens G, Leven D, Kelley M, Pennock B, Rogers R: The diffusing capacity as a predictor of desaturation in patients with COPD (Abstract). Chest 84: 327, 1983.

(61) Matthay RA, Berger HJ: Cardiovascular function in cor pulmonale. Clin Chest Med 4: 269-295, 1983.

(62) Robin ED, Gaudia R: Cor pulmonale: Including a short note on pulmo cordis (cardiac lung disease). D.M., May 1970, pp. 1-38.

(63) Yu PG, Lovejoy FW, Joos HA, Nye RE Jr, McCann WS: Studies of pulmonary hypertension. I. Pulmonary circulatory dynamics in patients with pulmonary emphysema at rest. J Clin Invest 32: 130-137, 1953.

(64) Lockhart A, Tsareva M, Nader F, Leblanc P, Schrijen F, Sadoul P: Elevated pulmonary artery pressure at rest and during exercise in chronic bronchitis: Fact or fancy. Clin Sci 37: 503-517, 1969.

(65) Butland RJA, Pang J, Gross ER, Woodcock, AA, Geddes DM: Two-six-, and twelve-minute walking tests in respiratory disease. Br Med J 284: 1607, 1982.

(66) McGavin CR, Gupta SP, McHardy GJR: Twelve-minute walking test for assessing disability in chronic bronchitis. Br Med J 30: 415-425, 1976.

(67) Kelley MA, Daniele RP: Exercise testing in interstitial lung disease. In Clinics in Chest Medicine, Vol 5 (No. 1), Philadelphia, WB Saunders Co, 1984, pp. 145-156.

(68) Boushy SF, North LB: Pulmonary function in infiltrative lung disease. Chest 64: 448-474, 1973.

(69) Fulmer JD, Roberts WC, von Gal ER, Crystal RG: Morphologic-physiologic correlates of the severity of fibrosis and degree of cellularity in idopathic pulmonary fibrosis. J Clin Invest 63: 665-676, 1979.

(70) Jones NL, Rebuck AS: Tidal volume during exercise in patients with diffuse fibrosing alveolitis. Bull Eur Physiopathol Respir 15: 321-327, 1979.

(71) Renzi G, Milic-Emili J, Grassino AE: The pattern of breathing in diffuse lung fibrosis. Bull Eur Physiopathol Respir 18: 461-472, 1982.

(72) Spiro SG, Dowdeswell IRG, Clark TJH: An analysis of submaximal exercise responses in patients with sarcoidosis and fibrosing alveolitis. Br J Dis Chest 75:169-180, 1981.

(73) Austrian R, McCLement JH, Renzetti AD Jr., Donald KW, Riley RL, Cournand A: Clinical and physiologic features of some types of pulmonary diseases with impairment of alveolar-capillary diffusion. Am J Med 11:667-685, 1951.

(74) Holland RAB: Physiologic dead space in the Hamman-Rich syndrome. Am J Med 28: 61-68, 1960.

(75) Hammer J: Cause of low arterial oxygen saturation in pulmonary fibrosis. Thorax 19: 507-514, 1964.

(76) McCarthy D, Cherniack RM: Regional ventilation-perfusion and hypoxia in cryptogenic fibrosing alveolitis. Am Rev Respir Dis 107: 200-208, 1973.

(77) Wagner, PD, Dantzker DR, Dueck R, dePolo JL, Wasserman K, West JB: Distribution of ventilation-perfusion ratios in patients with interstitial lung disease. Chest 69 (Suppl.): S256-S257, 1976.

(78) Carrington CB, Gaensler EA, Coutu RE, FitzGerald MX, Gupta RG: Natural history and treated course of usual and desquamative interstitial pneumonia. N Engl J Med 298: 801-809, 1978.

(79) Hoffman L., Cohn JE, Gaensler EA: Respiratory abnormalities in eosinophilic granuloma of the lung. N Eng J Med 267: 577-589, 1962.

(80) Sackner MA, Akgun N, Kimbel P, Lewis DH: The pathophysiology of scleroderma involving the heart and respiratory system. Ann Intern Med 60: 611-630, 1964.

(81) Davis JA, Frank MH, Whipp BJ, Wasserman K: Anaerobic threshold alterations caused by endurance training in middle-aged men. J Appl Physiol: Respirat Environ Exercise Physiol 46(6): 1039-1046, 1979.

(82) Hodgkin JE, Zorn EG, Connors GL: Pulmonary rehabilitation: Definitions and essential components. In Pulmonary Rehabilitation: Guidelines to Success. (Eds.) Hodgkin JE, Zorn EG, Connors GL; Boston, London, Sydney, Toronto, Butterworth Publishers, 1984, p. 3.

(83) Hodgkin JE, Branscomb BV, Anholm JD, Gray LS: Benefits, limitations and the future of pulmonary rehabilitation. In Pulmonary Rehabilitation: Guidelines to Success. (Eds.) Hodgkin JE, Zorn EG, Connors GL; Boston, London, Sydney, Toronto, Butterworth Publishers, 1984, p. 404.

(84) Karvonen M, Kentala K, Mustala O: The effects of training on heart rate: A longitudinal study. Ann Med Exp Biol Fenn (Helsinki) 35:307 -315, 1957.

(85) Exercise testing and training of individuals with heart disease of at high risk for its development: A Handbook For Physicians. New York, American Heart Association, 1975.

(86) Getchell LH: Exercise prescription for the healthy adult. J Cardiopulmonary Rehabil 6 (2): 46-51, 1986.

(87) Franklin BA, Hellerstein HK, Gordon S, Timmis GC: Exercise prescription for the myocardial infarction patient. J Cardiopulmonary Rehabil 6(2): 62-79, 1986.

(88) Hellerstein HK, Hirsch EZ, Ader R, Greenblott N, Siegel M: Principles of exercise prescription for normals and cardiac subjects, in Naughton JP, Hellerstein HK (eds): Exercise testing and exercise Training in Coronary Heart Disease. New York, Academic Press, 1973; 129-167.

(89) *American Heart Association:* Exercise Testing and Training of Individuals with Heart Disease or at High Risk for its Development: A Handbook for Physicians. Dallas, American Heart Association, 1975.

(90) Casaburi R, Wasserman K: Exercise training in pulmonary rehabilitation. NEJM, 1986 (Editorial, to be published). Also, Wasserman, K: Personal Communication, LAC-Harbor-UCLA Medical Center, Torrance, California.

(91) Borg G: Perceived exertion as an indicator of somatic stress. Scand J Rehabil Med 2: 92-98, 1970.

(92) Hage P: Perceived exertion: One measure of exercise intensity. The Physician and Sports Medicine 9: 136-143, 1981.

(93) *American College of Sports Medicine:* Guidelines for Graded Exercise Testing and Exercise Prescription, 3rd ed., Philadelphia, Lea and Febiger, 1986.

(94) Superko HR: Effects of cardiac rehabilitation in permanently paced patients with third-degree heart block. J Cardiac Rehabil 3: 561-568, 1983.

(95) Gordon NF, Kruger PE, Hons BA, Cilliers JF: Improved exercise ventilatory responses after training in coronary heart disease during long-term beta-adrenergic blockade. Am J Cardiol 51: 755-758, 1983.

(96) Laslett LJ, Paumer L, Scott-Baier P, Amsterdam EA: Efficacy of exercise training in patients with coronary artery disease who are taking propranolol. Circulation 68: 1029-1034, 1983.

(97) Pratt CM, Welton DE, Squires WG, Kirby TE, Hartung H, Miller RR: Demonstration of training effect during chronic beta-adrenergic blockade in patients with coronary artery disease. Circulation 64: 1125-1129, 1981.

(98) Hossack KF, Bruce RA, Clark LJ: Influence of propranolol on exercise prescription of training heart rates. Cardiology 65: 47-58, 1980.

(99) Chang K, Hossack KF: Effect of diltiazem on heart rate responses and respiratory variables during exercise: Implications for exercise prescription and cardiac rehabilitation. J Cardiac Rehabil 2: 326-332, 1982.

(100) Zack MB, Palange A: Oxygen supplemented exercise of ventilatory and nonventilatory muscles in pulmonary rehabilitation. Chest 88: 669-675, 1985.

(101) Shanfield K, Hammond MA: Activities of daily living. *In* Pulmonary Rehabilitation: Guidelines to Success. (Eds.) Hodgkin JE, Zorn EG, Connors GL; Boston, London, Sydney, Toronto, Butterworth Publishers, 1984, p. 175, 187.

(102) Criner GJ, Rassulo J, Celli BR: Respiratory muscle recruitment during unsupported and supported arm exercise in patients with severe chronic obstructive pulmonary disease. Chest 88 (No. 1; abstract): 14S, 1985.

(103) Leith DE, Bradley M: Ventilatory muscle strength and endurance training. J Appl Physiol 41: 508-516, 1976.

(104) Belman MJ, Mittman C: Ventilatory muscle training improves exercise capacity in chronic obstructive pulmonary disease patients. Am Rev Respir Dis 121: 273-280, 1980.

(105) Hunter AM, Carey MA, Larsh HW: The nutritional status of patients with chronic obstructive pulmonary disease. Am Rev Respir Dis 124: 376-381, 1981.

(106) Pardy RL, Rivington RN, Despas PJ, Macklem PT: The effects of inspiratory muscle training on exercise performance in chronic airflow limitation. Am Rev. Respir Dis 123 (4 Pt 1): 426-433, 1981.

(107) Sonne LJ, Davis JA: Increased exercise performance in patients with severe COPD following inspiratory resistive training. Chest 81: 436-439, 1982.

(108) Clanton TL, Dixon G, Drake J, Gadek JE: Inspiratory muscle conditioning using a threshold loading device. Chest 87:62-66, 1985.

(109) Weber KT, Wilson JR, Janicki JS, Likoff MJ: Exercise testing in the evaluation of the patient with chronic cardiac failure. Am Rev. Respir Dis 129: Suppl S60-S62, 1984.

(110) Rubin SA, Brown HV: Ventilation and gas exchange during exercise in severe chronic heart failure. Am Rev Respir Dis 129:Suppl S63-S64, 1984.

(111) Faulkner JA, Julius S, Conway J: Comparison of cardiac output determined by CO_2 rebreathing and dye-dilution methods. J Appl Physiol 25:450-454, 1968.

(112) Faulkner JA, Heigenhauser GF, Shork A: The cardiac output-oxygen uptake relationship of men during graded bicycle ergometry. Med Sci Sports 9:143-147, 1977.

(113) Bleecker ER: Exercise-Induced Asthma: Physiologic and clinical considerations. *In* Clinics in Chest Medicine, Vol 5 (No. 1), Philadelphia, WB Saunders Co, 1984, pp. 109-119.

(114) Anderson SD, McEvoy, JDS, Bianco S: Changes in lung volumes and airway resistance after exercise in asthmatic subjects. Am Rev Respir Dis 106: 30-37, 1972.

(115) Freedman S, Tattersfield AE, Pride NB: Changes in lung mechanics during asthma induced by exercise. J Appl Physiol 38: 974-982, 1975.

(116) Haynes, RL, Ingram RH Jr, McFadden ER Jr: An assessment of the pulmonary response to exercise in asthma and an analysis of the factors influencing it. Am Rev Respir Dis 114: 739-752, 1976.

(117) Kaplan AP, Natbony SF, Tawil AP, Fruchter L, Foster M: Exercise-induced anaphylaxis as a manifestation of cholinergic urticaria. J Allergy Clin Immunol 68:319-324, 1981.

(118) Lewis J, Lieberman P, Treadwell B, Erffmeyer J: Exercise-induced urticaria, angioedema, and anaphylactoid episodes. J Allergy Clin Immunol 68: 432-437, 1981.

(119) Sheffer AL, Soter NA, McFadden ER Jr., Austen KF: Exercise-induced anaphylaxis: A distinct form of physical allergy. J Allergy Clin Immunol 71: 311-316, 1983.

(120) Lim, VS, Zavala DC, Flanigan MJ: Basal oxygen consumption: A new technique for an old test. J Endocrinol Metab (in press).

(121) Lim VS, Zavala DC, Flanigan M: Hypometabolism in patients with chronic renal failure. Clin Res 32:269A, 1984.

(122) Lim VS, Zavala DC, Flanigan MJ, Freeman RM: Blunted peripheral tissue responsiveness in intact pituitary sensitivity to thyroid hormone in patients with chronic renal failure. (Submitted for publication).

INDEX

Dyspnea,
  differential diagnosis of, 46 (Fig. 9)

Ear oximeter. See *Oximeter.*

EKG,
  abnormalities, 34, 35
  electrode placement, 10, 11

Equipment. See *Exercise testing.*

Evaluation of patient, 6, 7 (Fig. 7), 8

Exercise team, 29, 30

Exercise training,
  of cardiac patients, 75-78
  of inactive older patients, 75-77
  of healthy adults, 76, 77
  of respiratory muscles, 85
  of upper extremity, 80
  of ventilatory limited patients, 79

Exercise testing,
  consent, 8, 9 (Fig. 2)
  contraindications, 6
  equipment, 12-28 (Figures 3-6)
  in asthma, 88, 89
  in cardiac impairment, 78, 87, 88
  in COPD, 72, 73, 79
  in interstitial lung disease, 73, 74
  in obesity, 89, 90
  indications, 5
  on the cycle, 31, 32
  on the treadmill, 22 (Fig. 4e), 23 (Fig. 5a), 24, 25 (Figs. 5b, 5c), 27, 31, 32
  predicted values,
    HRmax, $\dot{V}O_2$max, $\dot{V}_E$max, WRmax, 39, 40
  prescription, 76, 77, 78
  pre-treatment evaluation, 6, 7
  post-treatment evaluation, 35, 36
  report (data & interpretation), 49-53, 50 (Fig. 10), 66 (Exhibit 2), 68-71
    (Exhibits 3-6)
  responsibilities,
    of physician, 29, 30
    of technician, 30
  stopping the test,
    by patient, 34
    by physician, 34, 35
  type of test,
    constant load, 32, 33
    incremental, 33
    ramp, 33, 34
    steady state, 32, 33
    submaximal/maximal, 45, 51

P(A-a)O$_2$. See *Oxygen.*

P$_{ET}$O$_2$. See *Oxygen.*

Power,
 measurement of, 1

Pre and post test procedures. See *Procedures.*

Predicted values,
 HRmax, $\dot{V}O_2$max, $\dot{V}_E$max, WRmax, 39, 40

Preparation of patient,
 for exercise, 8, 10, 11

Prescription,
 for exercise, 76-79

Procedures,
 pre-test (by technician), 8, 10
 post-test, 35, 36

Protocols,
 for exercise testing, 29-36

Quality control, 91, 92

"R" (respiratory exchange ratio), 38, 43

Ramp,
 exercise testing, 33, 34

Rehabilitation, 75-79

Report form, 50 (Fig. 10)

Respiratory muscles. See *Exercise training.*

Respiratory status, 47

Responsibilities,
 of physician, 29, 30
 of technician, 30

Restrictive lung disease, 51, 64 (Exhibit 1), 73, 74

Rhythm disturbances. See *EKG.*

Riding the cycle. See *Cycle ergometer.*

SaO$_2$%. See *Oxygen, arterial saturation.*

Steady state. See *Constant load.*

Submaximal exercise, 45

Summary,
 of handbook, 93